THE PHYSICIAN WITHIN

THE PHYSICIAN WITHIN

Taking Charge of Your Well-Being

Catherine Feste

The Wellness Series
from
Diabetes Centers, Inc.
Minneapolis, Minnesota
1987

Editor: Michael Moore
Text & cover design: Terry Dugan Design
Typesetting: Associated Litho
Printing: Precision Graphics, Inc.

Diabetes Center, Inc.
Minneapolis, Minnesota
Copyright © 1987 by Catherine Feste
Published by Diabetes Center, Inc.
P.O. Box # 739
Wayzata, Minnesota 55391

Printed in the United States of America

Table of Contents:

Acknowledgements

Thank you to the following people for their contributions of mentoring, loving, believing, and generous sharing of themselves. I have dropped titles and degrees from their names. Beyond their knowledge it was their wisdom that guided me. Evelyn Anderson, Paul Batalden, Rich Bergenstal, Randi Birk, Helen and Paul Bowlin, Jo Bretzman, Anne and Paul Carlson, Bob Coniff, Norm and Ruth Dewes, Bob Donnelly, Maggie Duvall, Don Etzwiler, my family, Jack Fitzpatrick, Carmen Flum, Marion Franz, John Gerdes, Norma Goldberg, Sallie Gouverneur, Keith Gunderson, George Gura, Gustavus Adolphus College, Betsy Hedding, John and Donna Hill, Paul and Anabeth Hill, Bob and Lucy Hobert, Tim Hockin, Hudson, Wisconsin, Mary Jackson, Mel Jacobson, Dick Johns, Jerry Johnson, Dorothy Jones, Judy Joynes, Jim Klobuchar, the Lahls, Pat Lassonde, Steve Laxdahl, Leonard Mastbaum, LeAnn McNeil, Ruth Mitchell, George Molnar, Joe Nelson, Marilyn Nelson, Molly Pennock, Eric Petersen, Wendell Petersen, Carolyn Peterson, Ellen Reeder, Jim Reinertsen, Dennis Roof, Beth Ruml, Stephanie Dean Scott, Susan Showalter, Grant Sorenson, Dick Stahl, Judy Stephan, Maury Taylor, John Trelstad, Mary Lynn and Lee Tucker, Evelyn Young, and Jim Zetah. And special thanks to Mike Moore, who not only edited this book, but contributed greatly.

Expert Readers

I gratefully acknowledge the support of the following expert readers:

J. Paul Carlson, M.D.
Section of Oncology
Park Nicollet Medical Center
St. Louis Park, Mn.

Jaqui Duda,
a dear friend
and a true model
of the spirit of
well-being.

Roseanne Eschle-Smedstad, R.N.
Diabetes Nurse and Educator
Methodist Hospital, Minneapolis
President-Elect, American Diabetes
Association, Minnesota Affiliate, Inc.

Sharlene Jacobson,
an insightful friend
whose energy for living
and loving never ends.

Kathleen Kalb, R.N.
Coupled with the her professional
perspective is a personal vision
of surviving and living well.

Jim and Sharon Rendack,
two sensitive and
tenacious survivors.

Alice Ring, M.D., M.P.H.
Director, Division of Diabetes Control,
Center for Prevention Services,
Centers for Disease Control
Atlanta, Georgia

Audrey Rogness,
a friend well-acquainted
with The Physician Within
(it was she who named
the book).

And special thanks to Frederick Engstrom, M.D., Psychiatrist, Park Nicollet Medical Center, St. Louis Park, Minnesota, for his contributions to chapter 2, "Self-Image: Taking Charge of Who You Are."

For her wisdom, love
and never ending support
this book is lovingly
dedicated
to my
mother

Introduction

THE PHYSICIAN WITHIN is a literary rendition of its author. Cathy Feste developed diabetes when she was ten years old and discovered, as do all with a chronic illness, that it has a major impact on life. Some individuals become unaccepting, depressed, and disabled. Cathy was able, with help from those around her, to turn this experience into an asset. It was her attitude and determination that created her own "physician within." Through her numerous lectures throughout the country, she has joyously and unselfishly shared her attitudes and beliefs with others. She has truly enriched not only our local community and region, but indeed the entire nation.

Inevitably, generous givers receive more in return than they are able to share. For those who have not had the privilege to know Cathy or hear her speak, this book is truly a gift that will never stop giving. For those who know this vital, vivacious individual, and who are inspired each time we hear her speak, her book is an additional priceless gift that opens windows into our own lifelong pursuit of well-being. Cathy writes that it is impossible to know the true joys of life without knowing sorrow, because the most exalting sunshine is that which follows the storm. Never to be tested is never to know the joy of triumph. Cathy's thoughts and experiences, together with quotations from inspirational individuals, will create joy and a new philosophy of living for her readers.

We all know or have met individuals whose zest for life, whether it be quiet determination or dynamic enthusiasm, inspires us to pursue our own goals. Many of these people have discovered what Cathy has described as "The Physician Within." This book points the way to overcoming life's obstacles and realizing to the fullest one's reason for living.

For those with a disease or disability, it instills a positive approach to coping with what must be, while refusing to accept unnecessary limitations to one's goals and enjoyment of life. This book simply must be read by anyone who is angered or embittered by a disease or disability. It combines both a practical and an inspirational approach to changing one's feelings about oneself and about life. It helps build the self-confidence and the life skills everyone needs to enjoy real well-being, and which become even more critical when one develops a disease or disability. The book culminates in a description of a powerful healing and strengthening force each of us possesses, but which we must define for ourselves, develop, and invest with our sincere belief and faith.

The Plan of Action in the final chapter reflects Cathy's knowledge and conviction that it is not enough to read and talk about what we want out of life, we *must* take action. We must apply our knowledge, our life skills, our sources of support, and our motivation for well-being to define our goals and take steps toward reaching them.

Life has its difficulties, and these are not shared equally among us. Greatness is often a product of tempering. True greatness is not to be found in public fame, but in the capacity to be strong, inspirational, and loved by others. Cathy is such an individual and her book reflects that greatness.

Donnell D. Etzwiler, M.D.
Founder and Director,
International Diabetes Center
Minneapolis, Minnesota

For those interested in creation stories I offer this prologue.

The seed for this book was planted in 1957 when I was diagnosed as having diabetes. That began my personal excursion into well-being. My professional interest in well-being began in the early 1970s when I was the education director for the Minnesota affiliate of the American Diabetes Association. In that position I observed a great disparity among people with diabetes. Some became angry and bitter and sort of dropped out of life. Others took their diabetes in stride and continued to enjoy a fulfilling and enjoyable life. The difference did not seem to be related to anything physical. Some with the greatest physical problems had the biggest smiles on their faces.

My study began. My research question was: "Why do people do well?" I studied healthy people everywhere. They were "healthy people" who had diabetes, cancer, arthritis, or some other great life challenge such as the loss of a limb, spouse, or child. The common denominator was that they were all survivors. They chose to keep going instead of giving up. They chose to gracefully incorporate their challenge into their lives, neither making battle with it nor ignoring it. They didn't fit the popular image of "diabetics," "arthritics," "epileptics," or "cripples." They continued to be active, happy individuals who happen to have a health challenge.

The more I studied these people the more exciting it became. I observed some unmistakable common threads in the fabric of their lives. By weaving those threads together I developed a lecture-discussion series: Today Well-Lived. The lecture series became the basis for this book, which covers health challenges in general.

This book is about well-being . . . the unique well-being that people attain when they cope successfully with a challenge. I have not described every challenge, but I have described the process which I believe leads to a fulfilling sense of well-being no matter what your individual challenge might be. No book, person, or organization can tell you how to live well. Each individual must discover how to do that for himself or herself. What this book does is to take you through a process that will lead you to self-discovery. What I have done is to study, observe, apply, and evaluate. Do the same. Bring your challenge and unique personality and put them through the process described in this book.

Study the information and inspirational thoughts presented here, and use them as a springboard to applying them in your life. Seek other books on related topics, and take classes offered in these basic life skills. Observe how others use those skills. Especially observe successful role models around you. How do other people successfully cope with their challenges?

Apply the information you have gathered through study and observation to yourself. There can be no definitive answer to any of these complex life skills that will apply to everyone. Seek your own unique application.

Finally, evaluate. Was this new skill helpful to you? If not, study and observe some more. Find another insight into your challenge and apply it. Never stop studying, observing, applying, and evaluating.

This book has at least three possible uses. You may choose to read it and reflect onit alone. You may wish to use it as a guide for discussions with your various advisors. You may want to use any portion but especially the reflection and discussion questions at the end of each chapter as the basis for discussions in a support group. No matter how you use it, remember that the whole purpose is to improve your well-being.

The process of improving your well-being , like life itself, is a journey rather than a destination. This book was written to make your trip easier and more pleasant.

I know of no more encouraging fact than the unquestionable ability of man to elevate his life by a conscious endeavor.

Henry David Thoreau

Wishing you Well,
Catherine Feste

A Lifetime of Well-Being!

Some call it happiness. Others call it health. Still others generated a whole movement they called "wellness." What it comes down to is a general *good* feeling about life—a feeling of well-being. The question for many, especially those of us who must cope with a disease as part of life, is how to maintain a lifetime of well-being.

Each time life brings us a challenge—something that changes the way we need to deal with our daily schedule—we need to figure out how to maintain or regain a sense of well-being. Each of us defines well-being differently, but there are some elements of it that appear in the way most of us describe it:

Feeling in control of my life.
Having a sense of purpose in life.
Sharing life's ups and downs with friends.
Having fun.
Feeling good about who I am.
Being able to give of myself to others.
Doing meaningful, productive work.
Loving.

Many life events can threaten our sense of well-being. Losing a job or experiencing the loss of a major personal relationship can threaten just about all of the elements listed above. There seems to be an answer to alleviate these threats to well-being: get a new job, or seek a new relationship.

But what happens when you get a chronic disease? No matter how threatening it may be to your sense of well-being, a disease cannot be divorced or replaced. It *must* be made part of your life. The vital question is whether you succeed in making it part of an overall healthy life, or whether it overcomes your pursuit of well-being. Some individuals with a chronic disease would think this is a ridiculous question. There is an important difference among those individuals, however. Some think it ridiculous because being healthy seems out of the question once they get a disease. Others think it ridiculous because no matter what their challenge they continue to live with a healthy outlook. The latter is what this book is about.

Ultimately, well-being is an approach to life. You can choose to have a life of well-being. Even if you have a disease, you can still be a hearty, vital person. In fact, many people with diseases are more well than are their "healthy" counterparts. Well-being is not something you achieve in spite of suffering. It is something you attain because of suffering.

"Out of suffering have emerged the strongest souls;
the most massive characters are seared with scars."

E.H. Chapin

Read through the following two case studies. Identify the elements which make one a study of healthy attitudes and behaviors while the other is descriptive of unhealthy attitudes and behaviors. What suggestions would you make to change the unhealthy situation to a healthy one?

Sandy is seventeen years old. She has had diabetes since she was fourteen. She has not told many of her friends that she has diabetes. She does not want to be considered different from them. She understands what diabetes requires of her but she resents what she calls its "demands". So, sometimes she does not bring a snack with her when she is to be gone in the afternoon.

One day Sandy and a friend planned to go boating at the friend's lake cabin. Although Sandy prepared by packing sun tan lotion, towel, bathing suit and straw hat, she did not pack food either for her afternoon snack or for a possible insulin reaction.

Sandy and her friend arrived at the lake and immediately went out in the boat. They listened to the radio, chatted and sun-bathed. By 3:00 p.m. Sandy began to feel a bit shaky. She looked in her friend's cooler and found only sugar free pop. She was beginning to have an insulin reaction and she had nothing with sugar in it so that she could boost her falling blood sugar.

Sandy's friend had to quickly drive the boat back to their cabin where, fortunately, they had some sugar left from the previous summer. What if there had been nothing there either?

Sandy's response to this situation was, "That darned diabetes! It's always getting in my way. I can't have 'normal' fun like my friends do. I hate having diabetes."

Case study #2

Lucy is fifteen years old and has had diabetes since she was ten. She tells her friends about diabetes but she doesn't make a big deal out of it. She explains what she has to do and why, then goes about her life.

One day Lucy and a friend decided to go shopping. As Lucy planned her day, she brings money because she and her friend will eat lunch at the shopping center. Realizing that there is plenty of food available at the shopping center, Lucy reasons: "If I need a snack or something for low blood sugar, I can always buy something . . . but I should have something with me 'just in case' ." So, Lucy packs a small can of juice and a bag of graham crackers.

Lucy and her friend get to the shopping center by riding a city bus. Their shopping takes them to many stores and they do a lot of walking. At eleven a.m. they decide to take a bus over to a neighboring shopping center. There they will have lunch and shop a bit more before returning home. Just after boarding the bus, Lucy begins to feel lighheaded and sweaty. She's beginning to have an insulin reaction. Confidently, she reaches into her bag for her juice. She drinks the juice, then eats a graham cracker. As her friend joins her in eating a cracker she expresses here appreciation to Lucy for helping her to eat nutritiously.

By the time they arrive at the shopping center Lucy is feeling just fine again. Soon, they both forget about the brief incident with low blood sugar. Their memory of the day is that of fun.

Think of examples relating to your health challenge. See yourself in a social, family or work situation. Discuss why it is difficult to handle certain situations with positive attitudes and healthy behavior. Now, discuss how that situation can be handled with a spirit of well-being.

Living well with a challenge is really the thrust of this entire book. Life brings many challenges: growing up, getting a job, changing jobs, losing a job, getting married, losing your spouse, moving to a different part of the country, rearing children, caring for aging parents . . . and getting a disease, which is the challenge upon which this book will focus. Since challenges simply cannot be avoided, we must learn how to live well with them.

"Life is not a matter of holding good cards.
It's playing a poor hand well."

Robert Louis Stevenson

Stevenson reportedly had tuberculosis. His quote depicts a spirit of determination, which can guide each of us to live well with any challenge life brings.

The medical aspect of living well with a disease comes from the advice of a knowledgeable, skilled and caring medical team. A good team teaches clients the healthy behaviors to follow in order to control the disease or the effects of it. For you to be motivated to follow the advice of your medical team, you need to approach life with the attitude that you *will* live a life of well-being. One of the most important aspects of this attitude is the belief that life is worthwhile. Medical advisors can tell you *how* to live; you must supply the important *why*.

The essence of living well with your disease is your answer to these questions: Why do you want to live well? What is it that makes your life worthwhile? It is the answers to these questions, your *why*, that will motivate you to follow the *how*.

"He who has a why to live can bear almost any how."
Friedrich Nietzsche

Identify your purpose in life

Each of us has our own idea of what it means to live well. Broadly, you might describe it as your purpose in life. Ichiro Shioji, president of the Japanese Auto Workers, made this insightful observation: "For workers to find satisfaction in life and in the workplace, they must have a long-term purpose; they must have their efforts evaluated objectively and be rewarded for those efforts, and they must have friends around them." Although he applied this to productivity in the workplace, it surely has a broader application. Try substituting "well-being" for "productivity" in the following quotation:

"Productivity can be realized if you believe in the future, if you believe that today is going to be better than yesterday and tomorrow is going to be better than today

. . . then the productivity is there and that is expressed in Japan in having a meaningful purpose for work and for living."

Ichiro Shioji, in Automotive News

What does living well mean to you? To help you discover your own definition of living well, explore the areas of your life that you value the most. Some people break these important areas into the following: Work, Family, Social, Physical, Mental, and Spiritual. What is it that you value about each of those areas?

A friend of mine, a physician, told me about a patient of his who was dangerously overweight. After an absence of several years she made an appointment. She had lost 30 pounds since he had last seen her. He asked if she had discovered a new diet. She responded, "No, I've known for many years what I needed to do and how to do it. One day I was watching my children play and I realized how much I want to watch them grow up." Her children became her *why*.

Assess what in life is important to you. Those values can become *your* why, if you can succeed in focusing on them strongly enough. They will motivate you, inspire you, and sustain you through even the most difficult *how*.

Approach all challenges well

When people get a disease, the approach they take to the disease usually reflects their basic approach to life. Janet and Dorothy are interesting examples of this point:

Janet is a 37-year-old secretary. She has worked at a large insurance company for 15 years. One day she was told by her boss that she was being considered for a promotion. She declined the promotion, saying that she was really too old to get into something new, to learn all that would be required. She didn't think she could handle it.

There is nothing medically wrong with Janet, but she does complain of being tired most of the time, so she turns down many invitations from friends. Not only does she lack energy, she also lacks enthusiasm for hobbies, projects, her work ... even her family. Janet is not ill. But is she well?

Dorothy is a 50-year-old widow with three teenaged children. She works outside the home to support her family. She would prefer to stay at home, but she must work to help support her family, so she has chosen to make the best of it. She approaches her work with enthusiasm instead of resignation. She is looking into further schooling for herself, realizing that once her children leave home she will need to have meaningful, enjoyable, fulfilling activity in her life.

Within six months of one another, Janet and Dorothy both are told they have cancer. How do you think each responded to it? Which one thought of it as "the end of the world?" Which one looked at it as a "challenge that I can handle?" Which one used it as an excuse to not do things? Which one sought the best medical and educational advice so as to "get the best of it so it won't get the best of me?"

Two years later, Janet has transferred all of her negative feelings about life to her cancer. It used to be her "rotten job" that made her tired and irritable. Now it's her "lousy cancer." Even though her chemotherapy treatments cause her to feel ill only occasionally, Janet complains constantly that she doesn't feel well, doesn't have any energy, can't work, can't see friends, etc. Her lack of energy is blown all out of proportion in terms of what is caused by cancer or its treatment. Janet is undeniably ill, but so is her whole approach to life.

Dorothy is a sharp contrast to Janet. She gets the same chemotherapy treatments as Janet and they do zap her energy for awhile. Instead of complaining as Janet does, Dorothy adjusts her lifestyle to accomodate her low energy days. She fills those days with activities she can handle and does not complain about how she feels. On the days she feels well she functions absolutely normally. She shares her simple but beautiful philosophy: "I savor the good days and make the most of each moment when I feel well. I never look back at the days of illness. I only look forward to the activities I enjoy: seeing my friends, being with my family, doing my work, and giving to my community."

Dorothy and Janet have the same doctor. He feels very optimistic about Dorothy's chances of doing well but is concerned about Janet's future. Doctors have understood for many years that attitude plays an important role in healing. Dorothy's upbeat, forward-thinking, positive attitude will serve her well.

For Janet and Dorothy, well-being has nothing to do with a physical state of being. Long before each got cancer, each demonstrated her basic approach to life.

Dorothy's approach illustrates an observation many people have made over the years. Individuals who do well with any disease tend to have the belief that life is too worthwhile to give up just because they have a disease. When disease or adversity strike these people, they simply do not allow it to interrupt their life. Their desire to continue living a satisfying life inspires them to figure out how to work their disease into their life.

There is a frequently quoted statement which says that "Life is a journey, not a destination." The point is to make the journey enjoyable and fulfilling, no matter how many detours or roadblocks one encounters. Which elements constitute well-being in your life? Continue to make them your focus in life. If you have lost sight of these objectives because of a disease, now is the time to regain a sense of purpose. You *can* recapture the fulfilling life that may seem threatened.

When people complain that a disease has robbed them of a

fulfilling life, they need to examine exactly which elements of well-being are under fire. Although diseases cannot always be cured or even controlled, well-being can be restored. The diagnosis of a disease may seem to launch life out of control, but by understanding the disease a person can regain that important sense of being in control.

Friends and fun need not be abandoned because one has a disease. Self-esteem can even increase as the individual discovers personal strength never before tapped. A lifetime of well-being is well within your grasp if you make use of the life skills that comprise the remainder of this book.

The goal of this book is to help you work your disease into a satisfying, fulfilling life. To reach that goal in your life, you must understand and use the skills that work together to help an individual live well in spite of, and even because of, the major challenges he or she faces. Each chapter of this book describes one of those skills. But it is not enough to just read about them; you *must* apply them to your own situation and take action to make them work for you. The chapter summaries and reflection questions will help you apply ideas to your life and take action. Do them as you read the book the first time, and then come back to them as often as you feel the need to reinforce your resolve to live well!

Learn and use life skills

One important skill is developing and/or maintaining a positive **self- image**. Some people internalize their disease to the point where they define themselves in terms of their disease: they are an arthritic, diabetic, epileptic, etc., instead of regarding themselves as simply someone who happens to have a disease. The next chapter, "Self-Image: Taking Charge of Who You Are," promotes a positive and healthy self-image.

Motivation is a key element to healthy living. People know the type of foods required for healthy living, but they aren't motivated to eat that way. You may feel quite convinced that optimistic people do indeed do better than pessimistic people, yet you may not be able to find the motivation to stop giving in to the messages of gloom and doom so that you can start your journey toward hope. Chapter 3, "Motivation: Light Your Own Fire," looks at motivational theories and their practical applications.

Adaptability, discussed in Chapter 4, is another rung on the ladder of well-being. It is adaptability that will help you view disease as a detour and not a destination. When people adapt successfully to the changing circumstances of life, they find alternate routes that lead to their original and ongoing goal of a happy and fulfilling life.

Successful **stress management** is yet another important element. Stress can make most diseases worse, so it is crucial, even "medicinal," to manage stress well. Sometimes people choose destructive methods of coping with stress. A person with diabetes may worsen the disease by coping with stress by overeating. A heart patient may further compromise his or her health by coping with stress by smoking cigarettes. The examples could go on and on. The point is that you learn positive methods of coping with stress and use them. These issues are covered in Chapter 5: "You and Stress. Who is in Control?"

Chapter 6, "Insights Into Solution Finding" explores a step-by-step practical process for the important skill of **problem solving**. Important attitudes such as desire, determination, and perseverance are also discussed.

Social scientists have for many years emphasised that one of the most important aspects of a healthy life is **support**. Healthy people have the support of friends, family, neighbors, and others whom they identify as important. Beyond the general vital feeling one gets from having support, specific areas of life also benefit from the feelings of strength and reassurance we can get from others. Parents find support in talking with other parents about the challenges of child-rearing. "Mentoring," or sharing problems and successes with someone experienced in one's chosen field, is an important form of support in education and job satisfaction. And, when you get a disease, you need specific support from a knowledgeable and caring medical team, loving family, concerned friends, and from positive role models who have the same disease and live well with it. Chapter 7, "Getting the Support You Need," will help you decide what types of support you need and what methods you can use to get it.

Besides the external support you get from others, you have an essential source of internal support, which is described in Chapter 8: "Discover Your Physician Within." Everyone needs a never-ending source of energy, strength, and inspiration to bring them through the lowest points of life, to give them hope when the situation seems hopeless, and to give the support necessary to persevere and live well. Each of us has this source, and each of us must identify it and characterize it within his or her life. For many, the physician within is God or another all-powerful religious figure. Just as no one can decide what another will truly believe, no one can determine for you what the source of your inner support—Your Physician Within—will be. This book may help you identify *your* physician within. In so doing, you will develop and further your personal faith in the strength and invulnerability of your internal support, which you will then be able to call on no matter how hopeless things seem.

The final chapter is "Make Your Plan of Action!" In it, you will reflect on all the skills leading to well-being and construct your unique plan for achieving well-being in your life.

When you have all this in place, who could argue that you are not healthy? Some individuals will even be fortunate enough to be able to control their disease and enjoy a high degree of physical health. But *everyone* can achieve well-being of the spirit. Physical health may not be part of the Plan for everyone, but your approach to every challenge that life brings can be one of well-being. In that approach to life there is victory.

Summary

Well-being is something an individual attains by learning to live well with the challenges life presents.

The medical aspect of living well comes from being a part of a knowledgeable, skilled, and caring medical team.

Each individual places special value on certain things in life, and those values provide the motivation to live well. They are the "why" that makes it possible to live with any "how."

How an individual approaches living with a disease usually reflects his or her basic approach to life. A person who is committed to making the most out of life will be inspired to figure out how to continue to live well with disease.Skills that must be developed and continually sharpened in order to live well with a disease include: positive self-image, motivation, adaptability, stress management, solution finding, support from others, and internal support from a force that must be individually sought and defined, but that can be referred to as "The Physician Within."

A "Plan of Action" is a vital tool for using skills to achieve a personal file of well-being.

Not everyone with a disease can attain a high degree of physical health, but *everyone* can achieve well-being of the spirit.

Reflection Questions

1. Identify elements that describe *your* sense of well-being. Circle those below which apply, then add others if you like.

   Feeling in control of my life.

   Having a sense of purpose in life.

   Sharing life's ups and downs with friends.

   Having fun.

   Feeling good about who I am.

   Being able to give of myself to others.

   Doing meaningful, productive work.

   Loving.

2. Describe your purpose in life.

3. Describe your current greatest threat to your well-being and/or to your purpose in life. (Be specific in identifying which elements of your well-being or purpose statement you feel are "under fire.")

As you read this book keep focusing on both

1. Your definition of well-being, and

2. The threat you feel to your well-being.

As you read each chapter look for ways to *overcome* the threat and identify ways to *reinforce* your sense of well-being.

Self-Image: Taking Charge of Who You Are!

Self-image is a powerful force in our lives. How you *feel* about yourself has a great influence on how people react to you. Who you *think* you are determines what you do and how you feel about yourself. Negative self-image plays a major role in child abuse, spouse abuse, divorce, crimes . . . virtually all the failures of humanity. On the other hand, positive self-image drives people to emerge from ghettos to become community and national leaders. A positive self-image plays a large role in whether or not a person will succeed in life, and it also enables a person to nurture those around him or her.

One type of success that depends greatly on self-image is the ability to continue to believe in one's self-worth following diagnosis of a disease or developing a disability. Self-image is your armor, your defense against careless remarks, ("Oh, how long have you been crippled?"); ugly words and labels (deaf and dumb, spastic, arthritic, and diabetic); and the many negative messages that assault you daily. Self-image is also the powerful, positive vision which helps you not only to rise above the negative images, but more importantly, to gain self-confidence and to be at peace with who you are.

This chapter focuses on understanding the source and function of self-image and suggests techniques that can help you enhance your self-image and gain greater control over it. This will be a practical, down-to-earth approach to a highly complex issue. It starts with the premise that everyone's self-image can stand a boost.

For this approach to work, you must already have a fairly healthy self-esteem or sense of self-worth. If you have difficulty using the techniques in this chapter it may be that you need some professional help to "get the ball rolling." Evaluate yourself as you read and give the suggestions an honest try. If they don't help and your negative self-image won't budge, then you need more than this book can give you. You not only need more, you deserve more. Don't give up on yourself. Go to resources such as your physician, a family counselor, clergyperson, or a similar trusted advisor who can guide you toward getting the help you need to develop your positive and healthy self-image. Then, come back to this chapter for reinforcement.

What is your self-image today?

What words would you use to describe yourself? Put a check mark by the words in the following list that you feel describe you:

thoughtful	indestructible
self-confident	friendly
courageous	weak
generous	dishonest
assertive	honest
healthy	sickly
shy	trustworthy
fearful	a loser
successful	a winner

passive	unsure
loving	tough
attractive	caring
second best	ill
fortunate	tenacious
impulsive	out of control

Now, on a separate sheet of paper list your strengths and weaknesses as you see them. Remember that everyone has strengths. Be as generous with your self-appraisal as you would be in appraising a friend.

Did you find it easier to list your weaknesses than your strengths? If you did, you are in the majority. Most people do. Be sure that you have not short-changed yourself. You do have strengths. Make another list of the strengths that your greatest supporters (friends, mother, boss, neighbor, etc.) would say you have. These lists will give you some insight into your self-image.

This insight may or may not be an accurate description of who you really are. It is significant, though, because it is what you *think* you are. And what you think you are affects what you do.

People behave in a manner consistent with their self-image. For example, most smokers view themselves as smokers. In successful smoking cessation treatment using hypnosis, people are given the hypnotic suggestion that they are non-smokers. This has helped people to quit smoking. Their self-image has changed: Why would a non-smoker even buy cigarettes?

Hypnotherapy (the medical use of hypnosis) has been effective in changing other behaviors by changing a person's self-image. Overweight people find themselves losing weight when they cease to view themselves as fat, and instead think of themselves as slender—and eat accordingly. Self-image serves very much like a blueprint for behavior. That's why it is so important to have as positive a self-image as you possibly can.

Yesterday created today's self-image

One of the earliest and most significant influences on self-image is the message you got about yourself from your parents. Parents are like mirrors to which their children look to learn about themselves. By gaining parental approval, children gain self-approval. The message for a child is, "If my parents like me, then I must be a worthwhile person."

This concept is not universally understood. Some parents believe that if they give their children compliments and other positive feedback, their children will become egotistical and "spoiled". Thus, nurturing comments like "I love you", "I like you", or "You're a thoughtful girl," are withheld. This is unfortunate because it is those comments that develop a healthy personality and a positive self-image. Even sadder than withholding positive comments is the giving of negative comments like "You dummy," "You are so clumsy," "You lazy oaf," or "Hey stupid!" These messages of early childhood—both positive and negative—become the basis for a person's self-image. The actions of our parents also have a great influence on our self-image.

Our parents' behavior sends strong messages for our lives. If they tolerate cruelty, we abuse others. If they convey affection, we feel loved. If they demonstrate sloppiness, we never learn to take care of ourselves. If they limit our destructiveness, we learn self control. If they act courageously, we feel strong. If they are deceitful, we learn not to trust others. If they are active, we become partcipants. If they are hypochondriacs, we become sickly ourselves. If they make excuses for mistakes, we don't learn to control our own destiny. We *think* we are like our parents, and therefore we *learn* to live in the good or bad ways they demonstrate.

> Children are like wet cement. Whatever falls on them makes an impression.
>
> Haim Ginott

A person's self-image can be created not only by parents, but also by such authority figures as teachers, health professionals, and clergy, and by relatives such as aunts, uncles, and grandparents. Richly blessed is the adult who lived among nurturing adults while growing up. The healthy person leaves this loving environment of adult approval feeling so self-confident that he or she can take on the task of self-nurturing and approval giving. The positive self-image serves a function similar to that of a coach. When your parents are no longer doing the coaching and encouraging, you can look to your own internal coach for approval and advice. The person with a positive self-image finds a coach that *forgives* shortcomings (no one is perfect); *encourages* one's finest efforts (reach for excellence, falling short is better than not trying); and *loves* unconditionally (no matter what, you are a worthwhile person).

Children's minds are like tape recorders. They absorb what they see and hear and tend to believe indiscriminately all the messages to which they are exposed. Those tapes stay with you forever unless you challenge them and change them. A confident and capable executive confessed that he simply could not participate in the exercise portion of a wellness program. When we explored this with him he realized that his aversion to exercise went back to when his physical education teacher had called him a "klutz." Now, even as a mature and otherwise confident adult, he avoided exercise of any kind because he viewed himself as a klutz and was afraid of looking foolish. He was able to change that tape by replacing its message with one of his own: "I'm not going to let the careless remark of someone made years ago affect who I am today. I *know* I can exercise and enjoy all its fun and healthful benefits." Unless you take similar action to change your negative tapes, these tapes can continue to influence your self-image.

The world is indeed fortunate that the following people did not accept the messages they received:

* Thomas Edison was labeled "too stupid to learn."

* Grandma Moses was told she was too old to start painting at age 80.

* Winston Churchill was called "dull and hopeless" and flunked sixth grade.

* Walt Disney, who loved to sketch and draw, was told he had no talent.

* Louis Pasteur was rated "mediocre" in chemistry.

* Abraham Lincoln did not allow himself to wallow in these failures:

  1832-lost job and was defeated for legislature
  1833-failed in private business
  1835-sweetheart died
  1836-had nervous breakdown and was defeated for house speaker
  1843-was defeated for nomination to Congress
  1848-lost renomination
  1849-ran for land officer and lost
  1854-defeated for Senate
  1856-defeated for nomination for Vice President
  1858-defeated for Senate again

Other influences on your self-image appear in and throughout adulthood. Some of the early messages from your family will continue to be influential, in addition to new ones from co-workers, friends, social groups, clubs, religious groups, political organizations, and even comments and reactions from total strangers. Each of us has our unique culture that feeds us information about who we are. These influences of adulthood are reinforced by the tapes of childhood. The person who is overlooked for a promotion at work may respond:

from a negative tape by saying: "Of course I wouldn't get the promotion, I've always been a loser."

from a positive tape by saying: "Well, I must not have been suited to that job. If I keep doing the quality work I know I am capable of, I'll get another opportunity for a promotion."

In this way life experiences reinforce the old tapes and make a stronger case for one's self-image. The diagnosis of a disease can likewise be approached as either the natural outcome of a lifetime of rotten luck, or as a challenge that can be handled just as well as the previous life challenges you have handled.

Important and hopeful insight into human behavior and motivation comes from the world famous Menninger Foundation's Center for Applied Behavioral Sciences. At the heart of this remarkable center is this philosophy:

Your past is not your destiny.

We do not have to make the same mistakes, nor follow in the same life path and lifestyle to which we have become accustomed. We can make choices.

You control your self-image

No matter what your various cultures are telling you about who you are, you can choose the messages to accept and the ones to reject. You do this by changing the tapes—changing the messages you give yourself. You can change these messages by using one of the most effective mental tools known: positive self-talk. Mental health professionals call it "cognitive restructuring:" the changing of one's thoughts. The basic premise behind this tool is that thought creates feeling. You change the way you feel about yourself by changing your thoughts.

> The greatest revolution of our generation is the discovery that human beings, by changing the inner attitudes of their minds, can change the outer aspects of their lives.

> William James

The issue of aging has long been associated with this concept of mind-over-matter. We have all observed that those who stay "young at heart" seem to actually age more slowly than those who think of themselves as being handicapped by advancing age. George Burns, comedian, actor, and eighth wonder of the world, made a wonderful observation when he turned 85:

> Some people regard the age of 70 as old. They tell themselves, "I'm 70 and 70 is old. How should I act now that I'm old? Maybe I should sit down more slowly and walk more slowly. Perhaps I should even spill a bit when I eat." If these people practice really hard, by the time they're 75, they're pretty good at acting old. I'm no good at acting old because I never practice.

The important point is that George Burns refuses to accept the message given him by society. He altered his own attitude toward aging by giving himself positive messages like, "I can tap dance. I'm not old!" Negative messages tarnish one's self-image only if they are accepted as being self- descriptive.

Choose to reject negative messages

You cannot escape negative messages. The world is full of them. But you can choose to reject them. People who get diseases are sometimes "labeled" with terms such as arthritic, cerebral palsied, cystic, depressed, diabetic, epileptic, etc. You must view these labels as shorthand descriptions of conditions some people have, not as descriptions of the individuals themselves. You can help our society avoid labels by using appropriate descriptions yourself. Phrases such as "a person with arthritis," or whatever the condition may be, avoid the tendency of the listener to judge or think of the person solely in terms of his or her disease.

You can choose to take a negative message and reject it by using a technique that Dr. Albert Ellis, a psychologist, refers to as "talking sense to yourself." I talked a lot of sense to myself after the following experience:

> I was at a party, chatting with a man I'd not met before.

He launched into a lengthy description of his work. After a while he paused and asked, "What do you do?" I told him that I worked in motivation for healthy living and had gotten started in it because I have diabetes. Just as I was about to describe my exciting work, he interrupted me to say, "Oh, that reminds me of a paper I wrote in college, 'Sterilization of Defectives.'"

Using the technique of talking sense to myself, I rejected this negative message. I told myself, "Having diabetes surely does not make me a 'defective.' What a dreadful label! If there were a defective person in that conversation, it was not I." After talking sense to myself I did carry on to the point of getting a little spite, but I preserved my self-image as a healthy person. And, my own condemnation of the man's unfortunate remark became not the source of a bitter spirit, but rather a commitment to sensitivity and a caring spirit. That painful experience brought me growth. That's when illness becomes wellness.

Hold a psychological mirror up to yourself. Review the experiences you've had, the messages you've received, and most importantly, the messages you've chosen to believe.

Negative messages do not need to be dramatic to be destructive. They can, in fact, be quite unintentional.

At my clinic one day I gave myself an insulin injection with a disposable syringe. The nurse directed me to dispose of the syringe in a cardboard box in her office. When I looked at the box I saw the word "contaminated." I was startled. What was strictly a routine medical term became a negative insinuation for me. My message to myself to counter the inferred insult was, "I'm not defective and I'm not contaminated. I just have diabetes."

Negative messages do not need to be destructive if they are rejected and replaced by sensible messages.

Old negative tapes from childhood can be quite persistent in influencing your self-image. If you hear an old "I've always been a loser" tape playing in your mind, try starting an argument with yourself. When you hear negative self-talk, argue back with positive facts. Get your "coach" working for you! Here is how to have a healthy argument:

Negative: "Who'd want to hire a cripple?"

Positive: "I'm not a cripple! I may not move as quickly as I used to, but my mind is excellent and I'm honest, hard-working, and loyal. Who wouldn't hire me?"

Give yourself positive messages

Positive messages not only help to overcome a negative self-image, they are also needed to promote and maintain a positive self-image. "Daily affirmations" are one ongoing technique many have found helpful. An affirmation is a positive statement. Make a point of making a positive statement about yourself at least once a day. Just as it was a wise and loving coach who helped you argue with your negative self-messages, it is a wise and inspiring coach who gives you affirmations for encouragement.

A counselor with whom I worked not only recommends affirmations to his clients, he uses them regularly himself. In his office he has a sign that reads, "I am lovable and loving." It is only five words. It seems so simple. Yet it is a message that touches the heart of the human condition: our need to be accepted (loved) and to have the ability to love others. And, it promotes a healthy, positive self-image. If you have a hard time deciding on your affirmation, use this one.

Repeat your affirmation daily. It may take months before you begin to notice feeling more positive about yourself. Keep at it. The outcome is well worth your effort.

A woman with whom I worked once felt that her lack of patience was causing her great stress. Her frequent comments of, "I am so impatient!" only affirmed that negative self-image. So, she began giving herself a different affirmation: "I am relaxed. I am free of tension. I am patient." At a support group meeting several weeks after she began the positive affirmations, her husband remarked just how great a change he had noticed in her approach to daily tasks and annoyances.

The remainder of this chapter is a series of practical suggestions to help you develop a positive self-image.

Affirm Y-O-U

On the following page are most of the letters of the alphabet (X is missing). Following the letters are words of a positive and constructive meaning. Write your name vertically down the left side of the paper or on a separate sheet of paper. Next to each letter of your name write words that currently describe you or that you would like to have describe you. Using the word "capable" for the letter C does not mean that you are perfectly capable of doing everything. It means that you are capable in certain areas of your life. Everyone can honestly affirm that. For the C in my own name I would avoid words like "cold" or "careless." There surely may be times in my life I have behaved in such a manner, but an isolated event in one's life does not define a person's whole identity. Remember that. Forgive yourself what is past. Build a positive future with positive messages today.

A: able, abundant, accurate, active, adaptable, authentic
B: balanced, beautiful, beneficent, best, blessed, brave
C: capable, caring, character, chipper, compassionate
D: daring, debonair, decent, decisive, doer, distinctive
E: eager, earnest, effective, efficient, empathetic, energetic, expressive
F: fair, faithful, festive, fine, forthright, free, fun
G: gentle, genuine, giving, glad, good, grown-up, gutsy
H: hale and hearty, handy, happy, humanitarian
I: illuminating, important, improved, individual, industrious
J: jovial, joyful, judicious, just, jubilant

K: kind, kindhearted, knowledgeable, keen
L: law-abiding, leader, level, lifeful, liked, lively, loving
M: mannerly, mature, merry, motivated, mover, musical
N: natural, navigator, needed, noble, novel
O: obedient, open, optimal, ordered, orderly, original
P: pacesetter, patient, peacemaker, peaceful, pleasant,
   practical
Q: quaint, qualified, quality, quick, quintessential
R: radiant, ready, real, reasonable, relaxed, reliable, romantic
S: self-disciplined, self-respecting, self-reliant, silly, solid, soft,
   spirited
T: tactful, tenacious, tender, thankful, thorough, tolerant
U: ultimate, unassuming, unique, upbeat, useful
V: valuable, versatile, vigorous, VIP, vital
W: warm, well, wholesome, winner, wise, worthwhile
Y: young, youthful, yourself
Z: zany, zesty, zingy, zippy

Look in a dictionary for even more ideas of constructive, positive words with which to describe yourself. Now, taking the letters in your name, choose a word to represent that letter and to describe the *you* that you want to be and *CAN* be!

Positive behavior creates positive feelings

Now that you have a whole list of positive words describing you, take the next step of following through with appropriate behavior. Look at the words you've selected to correspond with the letters of your name, and ask yourself what behaviors would match those words. If you chose "caring" for the letter C, for instance, define the specific activities in which a caring person would engage. A caring person might volunteer some time at the local hospital or in a nursing home, visit a friend who needs a boost, or help a family member with a special project. Enjoying the caring feeling you get from the behavior you choose will persuade you to see your new caring self-image as real.

A woman shared with me how she overcame her

self-image as a sick person. She got busy helping other people. "When I help others I see myself as a healthy, coping, giving person," she explained. She has learned how persuasive behavior is. By behaving like a coping, giving, healthy person, she came to see herself that way, and so did the people around her. It is, in fact, what she had become.

Take charge through assertive behavior

When people behave non-assertively they frequently view themselves as a doormat—someone whom everyone else is free to walk on. That's a terrible self-image to carry into person-to-person encounters. Expressing one's opinions, ideas, and beliefs without undue fear of contradicting someone else or not going along with a group increases self-confidence and adds to a positive self-image. In their book *Your Perfect Right*, Robert Alberti and Michael Emmons define assertive behavior as:

"Behavior which enables a person to act in his/her own best interests, to stand up for him/herself without undue anxiety, to express his/her honest feelings comfortably or to exercise his/her own rights without denying the rights of others."

Assertiveness techniques are presented in Chapter 7, "Getting the Support You Need." Assertive communication is required to ask your friends, family, and medical team for the support you need from them.

Below is a sample of assertive behavior and its positive impact on self-image:

Marion's doctor told her about a new drug for her arthritis. From the way he explained it Marion felt that it sounded like an experimental drug which had not yet been thoroughly tested. Some people feel comfortable trying experimental medications; Marion did not. She asserted herself by saying, "That sounds to me like it is too new to have been thoroughly tested. What are my other options?" After her appointment, Marion rode the clinic's elevator down to the lobby. It was apparent that someone was smoking. Marion again chose to be assertive. She turned to the person smoking, smiled, and in a firm but pleasant manner said, "I believe that there is no smoking allowed on elevators. There is an ash tray just outside the door; if you wish to put your cigarette there, I'll be happy to hold the elevator for you."

The impact on Marion's self-image is quite evident in the self-talk she practices on the way home. "I'm so glad that I questioned that drug. I really felt very uncomfortable about trying it. The doctor appreciated my honesty and the appointment went very well. Not only did he advise me of a well-tested drug that he believes will help me, but I also had the distinct impression that our mutual honesty and clear communication enhanced our relationship. And I'm really pleased about the elevator incident. He immediately put out his cigarette, apologized, and even thanked me for saying something. I really feel good about myself."

Keep an affirmations file

Everyone should keep a personal file that contains affirming, uplifting, and otherwise positive notes. I've kept such a file for many years, on the suggestion of the prinicipal of the school where I taught. Put *your* name on the file flag and fill it with notes, letters, newspaper clippings, cards you've received over the years, and anything else that constitutes a positive message about you. Read through this file whenever your life seems a bit dreary. It will provide you with a wonderful shot in the arm! It is difficult to maintain a negative self-image when you read a note from someone that says: "Thank you for bringing your special love into my life. Your thoughtfulness was greatly appreciated." Stock your file with all those things that lift your spirits. I feel just about ten feet tall when I read over some of the cards from my young son. Each "I love you, Mommy" is a real spirit booster!

"God gave us memories so that we might have roses in December."

James M. Barrie

What a lovely thought that is. However, some people seem to find it easier to remember the thorns instead of the roses. So keep a collection of special thoughts to help you remember the positive parts of your past.

Remember, you are special

That is not an egotistical statement, it is a fact. Accept compliments when you receive them, because you deserve them. Avoid putting yourself down and never say, *"I am only."* *"You are YOU,"* and that's special because you are the best you in the world.

In the late 1970's King Carl Gustav of Sweden visited the United States. One of his site visits was to Gustavus Adolphus College. I attended the luncheon given for the King. It was held in the hockey arena and thousands of people were there. I noted that the King at one point straightened up and looked to one corner of the arena. I followed his gaze. There stood the food service director, Evelyn "the white tornado" Young and her team of college student servers. Within minutes everyone in the arena was served a piping hot meal. The King led the ovation as we all acknowledged her excellence in serving. Before leaving the U.S. to return to Sweden, the King presented Mrs. Young with a medal for her outstanding accomplishment. She was decorated by European royalty for serving a meal well!

My other favorite illustration of the importance of each individual is the following:

You arx important! You arx xxcxptional! Thx nxxt timx you think you arx only onx pxrson and that your xfforts arx not nxxdxd, rxmxmbxr this typxwritxr and say to yoursxlf: I am a kxy pxrson! I am nxxdxd vxry much!

Give yourself a pep talk

In *The Magic of Thinking Big*, David Schwartz encourages people to give themselves pep talks similar to a commercial. Like the exercise that encourages you to use words for each letter of your name, this exercise avoids boastful, bragging language in favor of simple, positive values that you hold. By writing and reciting this pep talk, you feel better and better about yourself as you affirm these values. You may wish to select some of the words from the name exercise to use in your pep talk. A brief example follows:

> (Your name), you are an adaptable person. That is an excellent quality. No matter what challenge or disappointment confronts you, you are able to adapt and regain balance. In the face of adversity you have demonstrated that you can be brave and even cheerful. You are compassionate and caring. You are a good friend to others as well as to yourself. You are doing well.

A friend of mine, a nurse, read Schwartz's book and wrote this type of affirming message for herself. She read it often in the days before an important interview and again just before it. She told me that she felt a real boost to her self-confidence.

Thank people

It will boost your self-image to see how grateful people are to receive *your* gratitude. Fill someone else's personal file of affirmations. Have you ever noticed that people who thank others a lot, and always seem to notice the good that others do, seem to be self-confident and have a positive self-image? Visualize yourself behaving in the same confident and generous manner. Then, follow your mental blueprint for action by doing it. Psychologists tell us that behavior produces feeling. Tell people "thank you," send letters of appreciation to your bank, service station, child's teacher, a store or restaurant where you received nice service; give generously of praise and thanks. It will do *wonders* for how you feel about yourself.

Daydream

Visualize yourself as you want to be. Call it daydreaming or fantasizing or having a mental rehearsal. These things are often thought of as a waste of time, but they actually help us to relax, they give us clues about our concerns, and they help solve our problems. In biofeedback, hypnosis, and meditation, daydreams are used and enhanced to help people with tension-related disorders such as smoking and headaches. People are encouraged to focus intensely on their visions, conjuring up all the sights, sounds, and smells that are integral to these visions. For example, daydreaming of being at a lake cabin, smelling the bonfire, hearing the seagulls, and seeing the beautiful shoreline helps recapture the feeling of relaxation enjoyed in that setting.

Our daydreams express our current problems. If we pay attention to them we learn about our obstacles, our troubles, and our preoccupations. They provide very useful information. Don't dismiss them.

As mental rehearsals, our daydreams are priceless. We can *visualize* our daily triumphs just as sports psychologists help athletes visualize their performance. Or we can carry on mental conversations to prepare for a crucial interaction, such as a job interview or a personal confrontation to resolve a conflict. Or we can play with a variety of solutions and scenarios to help us deal with upcoming events. (For example, dietitians recommend that we do a mental dress rehearsal before eating out, *seeing* ourselves eating appropriately.)

Take charge!

Keep in mind that as old as you are right now, that's how long it has taken for you to develop the self-image you have. It certainly will not take that long to move toward a more positive self-image, but the process does take time. Make use of the suggestions offered in this chapter. Seek help if you feel "stuck" in a negative self-image. Above all, *Take Charge!* As Eleanor Roosevelt so beautifully put it:

> "No one can make you feel inferior without
> your consent."

Summary

* Your self-image is who you think you are, and how you feel about yourself. A positive self-image is your armor against negative messages and a powerful force to help you gain self-confidence in everything you do.

* Self-image serves as a blueprint for behavior. If you honestly view yourself and act in a way you would like to be described, you will find that you have become that way and are viewed as such by others.

* Messages received in childhood from parents, relatives, teachers, and friends are powerful influences on self-image. These messages become "tapes" that are played in our minds unless we consciously take action to change them.

* An effective way of changing negative self-messages is to practice positive self-talk. Thought creates feeling, and by changing the way you think about something, you can change the way you feel, which will help you take positive action. Remember, your past is not your destiny.

* Negative messages are all around us. You must choose to reject them, and likewise choose which messages you will believe and make part of your self- image. You can be your own coach, arguing against negative messages with positive messages that describe the healthy you.

* Use daily affirmations—simple positive statements about yourself—to promote and build on your positive self-image.

* Keep a written and mental list of words that describe positive characteristics you have and some that you would like to have. Use those words as guides for your behavior, which will create the positive image you seek.

* Assertive behavior is an important part of a positive self-image. Being able to express your views and feelings affirms your right to self-determination and says that you regard yourself as an important person.

* Keeping an affirmation file of everything that carries a

positive message about you is an excellent spirit booster when things seem dreary.

* Remember that you are special. Even things you do that may seem insignificant, if done well, can affirm your specialness and add to your positive self-image.

* Give yourself a pep talk that is like a commercial for yourself. It will be reflected in your feelings and actions.

* Be generous in your praise and thanks to others. It will do wonders for how you feel about yourself.

* Feel free to daydream, visualizing yourself as you want to be. Daydreaming can both relax stress and help in solving daily problems.

* Take charge of improving your self-image. If you are unsuccessful, seek professional help to get started. For many, that has been the most valuable gift they have ever given themselves.

Reflection Questions

1. Go back to the list of possible self-descriptions in this chapter after you have practiced the techniques for improving self-image. Return to the list often. You will begin to see yourself in more of the positive descriptions.

2. List your strengths and weaknesses as you see them.

3. List the strengths that your greatest supporters would say that you have.

4. Where on the scale below would you say your self-image falls today? Place an X where you think your self-image is right now. Write today's date below the X.

POSITIVE				NEGATIVE
90	75	50	25	10

Below are several more self-image scales. For the next year turn to this page every three months and place an X where you feel your self-image is at that time and write the date below the X. Keep track of your progress!

POSITIVE				NEGATIVE
90	75	50	25	10

POSITIVE				NEGATIVE
90	75	50	25	10

POSITIVE				NEGATIVE
90	75	50	25	10
POSITIVE				NEGATIVE
90	75	50	25	10

5. Reflect on messages you have received from others:

My parents told me that I am:

At work I am considered:

My friends think I am:

My family would describe me as:

6. Using the self-descriptions listed alphabetically in this chapter, write a positive affirmation of you by stating "I am . . .

Motivation: Light Your Own Fire!

M otivation has two important applications within the context of living well with a disease. Motivation can be crucial in determining: 1) behavior, and 2) attitude.

Some diseases require that the individual take a great deal of responsibility for carrying out the treatment. Motivation is important in these cases because it helps assure that the person will follow prescribed healthy behaviors. These can include taking appropriate medications, eating according to the prescribed meal plan, avoiding allergens, stopping smoking, exercising, and performing various other therapies.

Motivation can also play a large part in producing and maintaining a positive attitude. Any disease or life challenge can make a person feel sad or discouraged. He or she may even give up hope of living a happy, fulfilling life. People need motivation to keep the flame of hope burning.

Motivation is a necessary element in virtually every area of life—from the mundane to the monumental, from cleaning house to taking charge of one's health and well-being. It might strike some people as odd that anyone would need an extra push to take care of their well-being. Odd as it seems, it's true. Studies of people recovering from heart attacks showed that those who made the most progress were pet owners. They took care of themselves, eating regularly and exercising, because that's what they did for their pets. They were motivated by their love for a pet.

There are many complex reasons some people do not take good care of themselves. They may include feelings of hopelessness, loss of control over one's life, and a lack of goals in life.

Hopelessness is a major obstacle

People will not be motivated to take good care of themselves if they believe that their situation is hopeless. This hopelessness is seen in such comments as: "My mother had arthritis and she ended up in a wheelchair. That's where I'm headed;" or "My father died of a heart attack at a young age. So will I"; or "I've heard that diabetes is the leading cause of blindness. What's the use in trying to beat the odds?" or "Everyone knows that cancer kills."

The feeling of hopelessness comes from such messages of hopelessness. The previous chapter discussed how you can change your feelings by changing your thoughts. That's the best way to fight hopelessness. To every negative message in the preceding paragraph you can argue back with the following positive message: "There is so much more known about my disease today. Each day brings more information and better treatments, with the possibility of a major breakthrough in research. I will learn all I can. I will seek the best medical support. I will do all I can to manage my disease. And I *will* manage my feelings by continuing to give myself positive, encouraging messages. I am doing well."

As our exploration of human motivation begins, remember to continue to build your positive self-image. Motivation is an exciting, essential quality of successful, thriving, healthy people like you.

The fields of business, education, and medicine all share basic elements of motivation: Value, Choice, Goal setting, Goal achievement, Rewards, Positive reinforcement, Perks, and Belief. These elements can also be applied to living well with a disease. As each is discussed, apply it to your life and situation.

Value

Value is the foundation of motivation. You will be motivated by those things in life that you value the most. In the first chapter, you identified what "living well" means to you. You focused on what makes your life worthwhile. Review those thoughts, because in them you define what you value. It may be your family, your work, your faith, your overall sense of well-being, or your tennis game.

Be aware of all the positive reasons you take good care of yourself. That's wellness. It is a very positive statement about life to say: "There are things in my life that are more important than my disease. I take care of myself so that I can function well in my job, enjoy my family and friends, and take pride in myself. Disease is not my motivator. Life and love of life are my motivators."

Choice puts you in control

When people feel they can make choices in their lives they feel more in control. The sense of being in control of one's life is motivating. In a classic article from the Harvard Business Review, Douglas MacGregor reported on the "Theory X, Theory Y" approach to human motivation. MacGregor reports that Theory X tells us that people won't be motivated. They have to be coerced, directed, told what to do. Theory Y, however, states that people will be motivated if they have input into decisions that affect them. It gives you ownership and helps you to feel more committed to doing something if you feel you made the choice.

When I was 14 I was at an appointment with a dietitian. I was a very timid 14- year-old, but I finally got my courage up to tell her, "I don't like milk." She replied, "That's too bad, because you're going to drink four glasses a day." Years later I found that not all dietitians take that approach. I was fortunate to find a dietitian who asked me about my likes and dislikes and my lifestyle. We discussed what my meal plan would be. She didn't dictate it to me. I felt more in control—and followed my meal plan more closely—because I was given a choice.

People must feel in control of decisions before they will be motivated to change behavior. Individuals will be more motivated to make healthy choices if they are convinced that the healthy choice will lead to a favorable outcome. Thus, the person who has had a heart attack will be more motivated to exercise, eat according to recommendations of the American Heart Association, and manage stress *if* he or she is convinced that those efforts will reduce the risk of another heart attack and increase feelings of well-being.

It is motivating to take charge of your life. Making choices helps you feel hopeful about a healthy future. There are no guarantees that a particular drug, exercise, diet, or any other treatment is really going to help. The therapy itself may not improve or even control your disease or illness. But the very act of carrying out the therapy yourself is an expression of faith and hope in your healthy future. Believing something will help, and then doing it faithfully, are two vital steps in taking charge of your life.

Sometimes people have been helped simply because they believed in the treatment or the person who prescribed it. This is called the "placebo effect." It is the mind, body, and spirit working together to heal the physical problem. The medical community attributes the recovery or improvement of some people to their belief in the therapist and the therapy, rather than the physical effect of the therapy itself. Dr. Albert Schweitzer, physician and humanitarian, called the placebo effect, "The physician who resides within." Choose a therapy with the help of a competent, respected, and trusted medical professional. If you feel good about the advisor, then you can take control by carrying out his or her advice. And, because you believe in it, your belief may activate the physician within.

The choice that is most important and available is the attitude you take toward your challenge. Remember that your attitude is created by your thoughts. Here is a lovely and inspiring story to encourage your own positive, courageous thoughts:

> Although Henri Matisse was nearly 30 years younger that August Renoir, the two great artists were dear friends and frequent companions. When Renoir was confined to his home during the last decade of his life, Matisse visited him daily. Renoir, almost paralyzed by arthritis, continued to paint in spite of great pain. One day, as Matisse watched the elder painter working in his studio, fighting tortuous pain with each brush stroke, he blurted out, "August, why do you continue to paint when you are in such agony?" Renoir answered simply, "The beauty remains; the pain passes."

Make healthy choices in both therapy and thought!

Goal setting and achievement

Goals are very important in life. They become your roadmap for getting to where you want to go. You cannot get from California to New York by simply "heading east." You must follow specific highways, or you could end up in an entirely different place than where you wanted to be. Likewise, the absence of specific goals can lead to great frustration. The presence of goals can lead to great fulfillment in life. Improved health and a greater sense of being in control of life can come from working toward clear and carefully defined goals.

Be sure that you set your own goals. Listen to the advice of your carefully selected advisors, then choose your goals. You are ultimately responsible for yourself. Your advisors can only advise you. You decide whether or not to accept the advice and whether or not to carry it out.

One of my mentors is Dr. Leonard Mastbaum, an endocrinologist at Mt. Sinai Hospital in Minneapolis. He has an interesting way of encouraging clients to set their own goals. In his wisdom he realizes that the only goal a person will strive to attain is the goal they have set for themselves. Dr. Mastbaum draws a continuum, a straight line with a zero at one end and a ten at the other:

0 10

He calls it a management continuum. The zero is symbolic of the fact that the client chooses to do nothing to manage his or her disease. The ten symbolizes perfection; that is, the client is willing to do absolutely everything that is recommended. After explaining this, he asks the client to choose how much he or she is willing to do to manage the disease.

Apply this concept to your situation. Make a list of all the behaviors you would do if you were following your physician's advice perfectly. Then decide how many of the behaviors you are willing to incorporate into your life. If your physician has recommended ten behaviors, and you decide that you are willing to do five, place yourself in the middle of the continuum. Then, have a very candid discussion with your physician about the consequences of your proposed behaviors. Depending on your situation, your physician may say that your goal is perfectly reasonable and likely to lead to a good outcome. Or, your physician may say that 50 percent adherence to the recommendations will likely give you a 50 percent chance of doing well.

Due to our human nature most of us are inclined to take some "leeway" in carrying out advice we are given. Look at your continuum and set a realistic goal for yourself. When unrealistic goals are set ("I'm going to do everything perfectly") people often fail to achieve the goal. If your first goal is unrealistic and you fail, immediately set a more realistic goal for yourself. Here is an example of "leeway" :

The plan for a person with a mending heart may include recommendations such as returning to work gradually, adding hours and increasing intensity of activity over a period of time, following a specific meal plan, having a regular exercise time, and practicing positive stress management methods. Perhaps an individual is doing quite well with all the recommendations except for some of the food restrictions. That may be the leeway he or she chooses. If red meat is not on the meal plan, he or she may choose to have it twice a week. It is important to discuss the possible consequences of this leeway with a trusted medical advisor. Then the person has the information needed to take charge of his or her life.

Guidelines for Successful Goal-Setting

1. Choose a goal that is important to you. You will be more motivated to achieve a goal that YOU have chosen rather than one someone else has chosen for you. To choose health-related goals, have an open, candid discussion with your health team. The goals they have for you and the goals you set for yourself ought to be headed toward the same outcome: maximizing the quality of your life. Any health-related goal is a team effort. You need your medical team's support and they need your cooperation. Keep communication open.

2. Goals should be *specific and measurable.* Instead of saying, "I want to lose weight," decide how much weight you want to lose. Ten pounds, for instance, is a measurable and specific amount, so you will know when you have achieved your goal.

3. Goals should be *time-dated.* "I am going to lose ten pounds," is a goal you could have for 20 years or more! "I will lose one pound a week for ten weeks" is an example of a specific, time-dated goal.

4. Goals should be *evaluated* regularly. If you did not lose that pound this week it may have been unrealistic for some reason or there may be an obstacle that you must deal with before you can proceed to attain your goal.

5. *Reward* behavior instead of results. Surely the resulting weight loss is a reward in and of itself. To keep you going, keep rewarding your positive behavior. Choose a reward based on some of the insights offered later in this chapter.

6. State goals *behaviorally* so that you can reward the successful completion of the goal-oriented behavior. "I will walk three miles four days this week" is a behavior you can reward. Reward yourself for exercising, even if it did not result in progress toward your over-all goal of weight loss. The reward will make it more likely that you will keep exercising, which will eventually contribute to your weight loss goal.

7. Keep *well-being* as your real focus, because that is our true over-all goal.

If you find you are not reaching your goals, discuss it with your medical team. It could be that you are not being realistic and need to set different goals. If you are reaching them, pat yourself on the back and keep moving forward!

Achieving goals is motivating because success builds success. In as much as it is possible, set small goals for yourself so that you can achieve them within a fairly short period of time. Set the next goal immediately, reach it, set the next, and so on. You will experience a motivational boost to your spirit as you continue to look forward to your next goal. And, you will experience a motivational momentum as you have one success after another.

Many diseases require behavioral change. This book cannot list all of them. Determine your behavior changes with the advice of your medical team. Then set goals for changing behavior in small steps, if that is appropriate to your medical needs. Your medical team may agree to gradual—but specific—steps for making changes such as: cutting back on salt to reduce high blood pressure, adding medications in stages for various diseases, losing weight to help control Type II diabetes, and building up to a recommended level of exercise to promote mobility in some types of arthritis.

People don't always experience success no matter how closely they cooperate with the recommendations of their medical team. Sometimes things happen which are beyond anyone's control. The disease may worsen. A particularly promising therapy may not work. At best, you can be philosophical about setbacks and disappointments. At worst, your disappointment can stop your good efforts and darken your hope. Frustration is a major obstacle to motivation when it gets so far out of hand. This frustration stems from the natural feeling that your efforts should be rewarded. And indeed, they should. Your reward might not always be a positive health outcome, but it is important that your efforts be rewarded in some significant way.

Reward is a motivator

In 1912, Stacy Adams proposed what is called the Equity Theory of motivation. Adams said that everyone has a sense of fairness, and if treated fairly, people respond by working that way. Adams' observation describes a feeling that seems quite common in the United States of America. In this nation of free enterprise we are rather accustomed to receiving rewards in a direct relationship to how hard we work. "Work hard and you will be rewarded" has been a national expectation throughout our history. It appeals to a sense of fairness that Adams says most people share.

Therefore, it strikes people as *unfair* when they follow closely the recommended medical regimen only to find little or no improvement in their condition. They feel cheated out of a reward for their efforts. A person with cancer that does not respond to painful treatments may be aware of someone with the same cancer who *is* responding to treatment. That isn't fair, but unfortunately it is the nature of medicine: everyone responds a bit differently to therapy.

Likewise, a person with arthritis may say, "Esther and I got arthritis at about the same time five years ago. Today she's walking and I can hardly hobble. It isn't fair!" Or, "My neighbor Harry smokes more than I do and is even more overweight. How come I had a heart attack? It isn't fair!" Of course it isn't fair. It isn't that you would wish that these individuals were afflicted instead of you. It's just that you would like to be as fortunate as they. There is no magic answer to relieve the frustration and anguish that we can feel in these situations. Life simply isn't fair. We want it to be. But it isn't.

Since a positive outcome is not a guaranteed reward, you *must* develop other systems for receiving awards.

Rewards are particularly effective motivators when the objective is to change behavior. In the business world it is called "incentive motivation." But what it boils down to is this: When you get a reward for doing something, you are more likely to do it again. Behavior that is rewarded is repeated. This motivation technique is used in toilet training for children, obedience training for dogs, coaching athletes, and supervising employees. There is no reason it can't be used just as effectively for self-motivation!

In general, motivation by reward is most effective when used to achieve short- term goals. Getting your reward quickly will help in the early stages of beginning a behavior change. And especially when attempting to change a long- standing habit, you need regular, frequent rewards along the way to keep you going. For this reason, it is important to: *Reward behavior— Not Results*.

Let's look at weight loss as an illustration of this point. For a variety of reasons weight loss can be a very slow process. If you were to wait until you'd reached your desired result of, say 30 pounds, before you rewarded yourself, you would have a very long wait. The lack of a reward during that time will serve as a reminder that you have not succeeded, or perhaps are not even making good progress. The resulting frustration could lead to discouragement and giving up. The answer is to reward yourself for the positive behaviors of following your special meal plan, exercising, and avoiding situations that you associate with overeating.

Fred wanted to change his behaviors to achieve a more consistent lifestyle. Long business lunches and sleeping in on weekends were interfering with the exercise program designed to strengthen his mending heart. He set a goal of allowing no more than one lunch per week to interrupt his exercise, and he set another goal of sleeping in no more than one extra hour on weekends. He kept track on his calendar of how he was doing. Then, on the 15th and 30th of each month, he checked to see how he'd done. His reward for following positive behavior was to buy tickets to a baseball game, an extra afternoon of golf, or a professional shoe shine (something he really enjoyed but considered to be a bit extravagant—a perfect reward!).

Each individual must decide on his or her own rewards, because they must be things that truly appeal to you. Rewards need not be expensive. An afternoon at the art institute or a day spent browsing through a shopping center may be perfect. These rewards may require family cooperation if you need a babysitter while you're gone. Be creative. Make a list of all the possible rewards you could give yourself. Keep the list handy . . . you'll need it!

To help you get started on your own list of rewards here is but a beginning:

> a leisurely bath by candlelight with music
> a new book and time set aside for reading it
> an hour to listen to music you especially enjoy
> new make-up or a hair appointment
> tickets to a favorite event

special time together with a friend
a walk through a community rose garden
a small gift to yourself: a scarf, belt, cologne
extra time to spend on a favorite hobby
a brief vacation or trip
an extended vacation if you can afford it!
a telephone conversation with a special friend
that class you've always wanted to take
go on with your list . . .

Receive a double benefit from your reward by reminding yourself as you enjoy it, that you have earned it! Tell yourself that you are a winner and get daydreaming about your next reward!

Positive Reinforcement

Wouldn't it be wonderful if you had a cheerleader to follow you around giving you messages of encouragment and enthusiastically congratulating you everytime you did well? Parents, teachers, and other authority figures play important roles as "cheerleaders" for children. But adults need that boost too! A psychiatrist friend of mine said once that people need encouragement like plants need water. Humans have "recognition hunger." People like to receive recognition: everything from a simple hello from a friend to an award for an outstanding accomplishment. That's positive reinforcement. Motivation experts such as Frederick Herzberg, a businessman, point out that positive reinforcement is one of the greatest motivators known. Because it fulfills our hunger for recognition, positive reinforcement motivates us to repeat the behavior.

An amusement park instituted an incentive motivation program for their young employees. Customers were given cards that read: "Nice going!" They were asked to please give a card to any of the park employees who were especially helpful or courteous. The plan was to have the employees turn in their cards at the end of the season for cash or prizes. The park's customers not only willingly handed out the cards, they also wrote personal messages on them: "Dear Vicki, thank you for being so nice to our family. You made our day!" To the surprise of park officials, the young people didn't turn in their cards. The kind words—the positive reinforcement—were considered a greater reward than cash or prizes.

Fortunate is the person whose family, friends, and medical team give positive reinforcement for his or her healthy behaviors. Even if you do not have those people cheering you on, you can train your internal coach to give you positive reinforcement.

Dr. David Campbell, coauthor of the Strong-Campbell interest inventory, lectured once on motivation and advised this type of self-coaching. He told of a very motivated salesman he'd met. The salesman described how he coaches himself with positive comments. A sign in his garage gives him positive reinforcement every time he arrives home. The sign reads, "Welcome home, Olson. Well done!"

Train your coach by first listening to the messages you give yourself. Are they positive ("Nice going Mary!") when you succeed, and generous ("That's okay, you'll do better next time") when you don't succeed? Do you accept the positive messages and compliments of others? ("Thank you, I'm so pleased you like it!") Or do you throw compliments away? ("What, this old thing?") Fire a negative coach. Train your coach to be helpful to you by giving you only positive and constructive messages.

Another motivating aspect of positive reinforcement is that you receive a real boost when you give positive reinforcement to others. This boost is spirit-lifting! Most agree that people are more likely to be motivated when they're feeling *up* rather than down. Industrial psychologist Dr. Robert Hobert, of Minneapolis, Minnesota, states that through their behavior, people have a great deal of control over whether they feel up or down. Behavior creates feeling, thus giving out reinforcement makes people feel "up." A program Hobert presented to a major brokerage house was entitled, "How to stay up in a down market." His message was, "Give out positive reinforcement." This includes smiles, winks, handshakes, hugs, sincere compliments, any positive communication that positively reinforces another person.

The best way for you to learn about this is to try it for yourself. I tried it at the supermarket one day and the experience left me glowing:

> One day I was grocery shopping and I asked the produce manager if he had any fresh spinach. He asked me to wait while he went to the back room to get it. He returned with a bag of spinach. Then he carefully and courteously explained how I should wash it in cold water and drain it on paper towels. I thanked him.

> As I made my way through the store I saw a man who looked as if he might be the manager. A voice inside me said, "Practice what you preach, Catherine. Go tell that store manager what a nice produce manager he has." So I approached him and asked if he were the store manager. He instantly took a defensive posture and said suspiciously, "Yes?" I then said, "Well, I just wanted you to know that your produce manager makes it a pleasure to shop in your store. He is helpful and courteous, and I just wanted to thank you." The store manager beamed a proud smile and thanked me!

What a positive feeling I received from that experience. Create your own positive feelings by giving out positive reinforcement to the people in your life. Work at doing it every day until it becomes a habit. You will enjoy a continual uplift from the practice!

Perks

A similar suggestion comes from the well-known motivation

expert, Zig Ziglar. He compares motivation to the fire in a fireplace. He says that when the flames die down and all you have are glowing embers in the grate, you must take a poker and poke the logs. This usually results in a return of the flames. According to Ziglar, "That's motivation." He asserts that we are all smoldering embers inside. We need some external "poker" to give us a jab and get us excited again—to get those juices flowing and toes tapping. It is life's pokers that renew and energize and remind us how good it is to be alive!

Who or what are the pokers in your life? Make a list of the people, places, and experiences that energize you. Your people list might include friends who make you laugh ... acquaintances who are really turned on by life and who make you feel excited everytime you talk with them ... people whom you greatly admire and who inspire you through their conversation, books, lectures, or sermons. Your places list might include the inspiration of the mountains or the serenity of a quiet local creek. Your experiences list is truly boundless and might include attending the symphony or the local high school's production of a musical, singing in your favorite group, spending a weekend at a lake cabin, or watching a gorgeous sunset with a friend who enhances your enjoyment by sharing the experience with you.

Occasionally in life there occurs a truly "mountaintop experience." When you have such an outstanding experience, it serves as a poker while you experience it and then continues to give you a boost as long as you retain the memory. I had such an experience when I heard the wonderful Maria von Trapp speak. She is the woman about whom "The Sound of Music" was written. She described her philosophy of life as being described quite well by one of the songs from the movie:

"A bell is not a bell until you ring it.
A song is not a song until you sing it,
and love was not meant in your heart to stay.

Love is not love until you give it away."

I still get shivers every time I remember that glorious woman with her tanned, deeply lined, gracious old face, speaking those words so clearly and proudly. It will serve as one of my pokers as long as I can recall that scene to mind.

Perks are an expression of the rewards given by corporations to their employees for a job well done. You can take charge of the perk-giving in your own life! Make a list of all the perks you can possibly give yourself. Consider these perks your "resources for renewal" and go to them often. The time to think about getting yourself "up" is on a regular basis, not when you're so far down that it's really difficult to get back up again. Take a moment right now to begin your lists of pokers and perks:

PEOPLE   PLACES   EXPERIENCES   PERKS

Belief

Belief is the most powerful motivator of them all. You will not be motivated to do anything unless you *believe* that it will lead to a positive outcome. This is the simplest aspect of belief as a motivator. People who believe that aspirin will relieve their aches and pains are motivated to take it.

Another behavioral aspect of belief as a motivator is that people act according to their most dominant thought. In other words, people's behavior reflects what they believe in. One of the most dramatic examples I have seen of this comes from a man who participated in a seminar for people with diabetes. As I was teaching the seminar I noticed a man sitting in the back of the classroom who seemed very angry. He never participated in any of our discussions. He simply glared and frowned throughout the class.

After the third class, he approached me when everyone else had gone. He said: "Anyone who has diabetes and doesn't admit he's inferior is a G.D. liar!" I asked him how he had been told that he had diabetes. That crucial introduction strongly influences what one believes. He replied, "Well, I was ten years old and my mother and my doctor sat me down and said, 'You are sick. You can't go out for sports anymore or play with your friends the way you do now, because you're sick now.'"

Having been influenced in this way by these authority figures in his life, he believed that having diabetes meant that he would have to give up all the fun things in life. By the time I met him he had spent over 20 years believing that he was sick and that his life could never be fulfilling. He was living his life according to his most dominating thought: illness.

I couldn't help but think of the sharply contrasting situation in my experience with diabetes. I too was ten years old when I got diabetes. Daddy had died suddenly of a heart attack ten months before I was diagnosed. When my mother came into my hospital room the doctor had just told me that I have diabetes. I asked her, "What does it mean?"

With a big smile on her face, my magnificent mother said,

"Why, it means that we're going to learn so much about good nutrition. We're going to live such a healthy lifestyle that our whole family will benefit. And you will always be a stronger, more disciplined person because you have diabetes."

She had me sold! I wanted to go back to school and give it to my friends! Her positive belief, given with such conviction, became my belief. The experience shaped my life. It has helped me to act according to that dominant thought: wellness.

Motivation experts describe yet another aspect of the motivational power of belief with the statement: Expectation becomes self-fulfilling prophecy. This concept is illustrated in the following examples:

> The father of an acquaintance of mine comes from a family in which none of the men have lived beyond the age of 55. As this man approaches his mid- fifties, what do you suppose he's doing to preserve his health? Nothing. He smokes three packs of cigarettes a day and drinks to excess. He expects to die young. He is acting in a manner to bring that expectation to a self-fulfilled prophecy.

When my wonderful brother Pete was 38 years old he had a heart attack. It was, of course, shocking and difficult for all of us who love him. My first thought was for Pete's recovery and future well-being. Understanding the concept of expectation and belief, I was concerned that Pete's expectation for his future be positive. Daddy was 42 when he died of a heart attack. How easy it would have been for Pete to resign himself to a premature death. To encourage Pete's spirit of determination, I gave him Norman Cousin's book, *Anatomy of an Illness*. He loved it. It lifted his spirits greatly.

Then, I arranged for Pete and his wife to attend a weekend wellness retreat where he would gain information on living well. One of the important messages he got was that although heredity is certainly a risk factor in heart disease, virtually every other risk factor was something he could do something about. A combination of factual information, loving support and Pete's own determination and love for life helped him to choose a positive expectation. With hope in his healthy heart, Pete changed his lifestyle. His cholesterol has dropped significantly; he's a trim runner of 20 miles per week, and he feels wonderful.

I know that Pete genuinely believes in his healthy future. When he turned 40 he had braces put on his teeth!

Please do some careful self-examination at this point. What are your beliefs about your health challenge, and more importantly, about your future well-being? The Health Belief Model states that in order to take positive action toward health, people need three things: they need to understand the seriousness of their disease, they need to believe that they are personally vulnerable, *and* they must have a strong hopeful belief that they can do something to positively affect the outcome.

One of the most important things you can do to affect a positive outcome for yourself is *believe* in a positive outcome. It is very challenging to believe in a positive future when you are surrounded by negative messages about your future. During national diabetes month each year I find it challenging as a person with diabetes to remain positive and believe in my healthy future when I read billboards telling of the blindness, kidney failure, and heart attacks so closely associated with diabetes. At times it is extremely difficult to believe . . . but it is possible to do so.

Jackie Townsend provides a remarkable example of the power of positive belief. I heard Jackie, a former Miss America, speak several years ago. After her reign, she married and had a son and then a daughter. One night she awakened to hear her infant daughter crying. She tried to go to her baby but could not move. She was totally paralyzed. She tried to tell her husband that she needed help. She couldn't speak. At the age of 28 she had suffered a massive stroke. She spent the next years learning all over again to walk and talk.

Jackie had tremendous family support and still does. She told us that the only residual impact of her stroke is that when she becomes emotional, her words don't always come out. She told us that recently she was scolding her son, now a teenager. Suddenly, the words stopped coming. Her son waited a moment, then enthusiastically cried out, "Come on, Mom, you can do it!"

Two older women were sitting in front of me. One turned to the other and said, "Well, that's youth!" I disagree: *That's belief!* Jackie refused to believe the messages surrounding her about stroke "victims" and the "vegetables" they become. She replaced those negative messages with positive messages such as, "Jackie, you're 28 years old, you've got two babies, and you're going to make it." She believed in the positive outcome she ultimately achieved.

There are two tools you can use to increase your belief: 1) positive self-talk, and 2) visualization. Jackie Townsend's story illustrates the power of positive self-talk. The previous chapter on Self-Image described this technique. Use it. Definitely make use of it anytime you hear a negative message in your head. Replace those messages with positive ones. But use the technique in a preventive manner as well. On a daily basis give yourself positive "I can" messages. Examples include: "I am well." "I can cope." "I am getting better all the time." Make up your own messages so they are specific to your situation and your feelings.

Don Gambril, U.S.A. swim coach for the 1984 Olympics, says that the minute his swimmers begin to think negatively, their performance slips. So, to encourage positive thinking, he gives the swimmers cassette tapes to listen to. The tape's message is: "I feel great. The more I swim the better I feel. Replace *your* negative tapes with positive ones!"

Visualization

Visualization is a mental image or picture. To increase your positive belief, get a picture in your mind of yourself looking healthy. If you are to be well you must visualize yourself well. That mental image is a powerful motivational tool.

A futurist whom I heard speak at a long-range planning meeting once made the observation that no nation, corporation, or individual can hope to move forward positively without a belief in a positive future. He called this a "positive future self-image." *That* is what you must visualize: your positive future self-image. And then you must believe it. Logic sometimes does battle with intuition, making it very difficult to believe a visualized image. However, intuition will be more powerful than logic in persuading you and causing you to believe.

The brain has two hemispheres, the left brain and the right. The left brain is the side that views things logically. The right side views things intuitively. Some people tend to be more logical and others more intuitive. For those most heavily influenced by logic, it may be difficult to be intuitive and to believe in anything not actually seen. To encourage the intuitive side of yourself think of times you've actually seen the effect of the mind on the body. (Such as when you feel a cold coming on but you decide you're too busy to get sick, and at bedtime you visualize yourself at work the next day, busy, energetic and *well*. Or times when someone challenged you by saying you couldn't do something, and you *decided* that you could do it, and you did.) Recalling actual examples is a way of combining logic and intuition. You believe because you've seen. With time and practice you will believe after seeing it only in your mind.

One of the most common general uses of visualization is in sports. For years coaches have told their athletes, "Before you perform, *see* yourself doing it!" Thus, basketball players visualize balls swishing through baskets before they actually shoot. Golfers "see" their golf balls land on the green before they actually hit the ball. Dr. Denis Waitley provides an excellent golf illustration:

> Waitley worked with returning P.O.W.s from Vietnam. He tells the story of George Hall, who, before he went to Vietnam, was a semi-professional golfer with a handicap of 4. Hall was captured in Vietnam and placed in solitary confinement for five-and-one-half years. To keep his sanity he played golf mentally. Each day he visualized himself on a golf course and he watched himself golf stroke by stroke all 18 holes. When Hall finally returned to the U.S.A., within one week he played in the New Orleans Open and shot a 76. A member of the news media, aware of Hall's history, rushed over to him and asked how he explained his good luck. "Luck!?" exclaimed Hall, "I haven't had to 3-putt a green in over five years!"

Visualization works if it is supported by belief. I had lunch with a corporate president one day as we planned a motivational program for his employees. He told me that he was playing golf after lunch. Without explaining the concept I merely suggested to him that he visualize where he wanted each shot to go before he hit it. He said he'd try it. When I got to his company several weeks later the first question I asked was about his golf game and visualization. "It didn't work," he told me. However, after I gave my presentation and explained the importance of belief he rushed up to me exclaiming, "That's it! I visualized. But I didn't believe. I said to myself, 'That's where I want it to go, but it won't.'" Visualize *and* believe.

As you read this, remember the perspective from which I am writing it: Diabetes. Diabetes is perhaps the most patient-controlled of all diseases. Medications play a role, but only if the patient takes them appropriately. The meal plan, blood glucose monitoring, exercise, and stress management are left almost entirely for the patient/client to perform and interpret. People with diabetes need to be motivated to do all of the required self-care. I am convinced that to be sufficiently motivated, people must believe there is hope in a positive outcome. That positive outcome might be a remarkably healthy body 50 years after diagnosis. Or, it may mean that the degenerative blood vessel complications occur more slowly. The key is belief.

Treating some other diseases requires far less direct patient involvement. Motivation for behavioral change is less of an issue to these folks. When a change in behavior is not as likely to affect outcome, we concentrate on changing attitude. Since the mind, body, and spirit do affect one another, we need to stay upbeat and optimistic and provide a healing environment within our body. If healing is possible, we must believe that it *will* happen. It is then that the mind and spirit can participate in physical healing.

The healing power of belief is at best controversial. In the New Testament, Jesus is called the great Physician and repeatedly performs miraculous healing. A frequent quote is Jesus telling someone "Your faith has made you well." There are people today who believe that faith will make them well. There are those who say that is all "hooey." I believe in a stance which lies between those two extremes. I feel that faith is a tool to use along with conventional therapy. Faith in and of itself might heal . . . but then it might not. No one should feel guilty if they try techniques of belief or faith and do not get a positive outcome. It isn't because you "didn't pray hard enough" or "didn't believe strongly enough." It simply wasn't meant to be. Sometimes antibiotics help and sometimes they don't. But they cannot possibly help if we don't use them. So, try all the tools of healing: medication and therapies recommended by your respected medical team as well your own positive belief.

One more thought about positive outcomes is that we can greatly expand the definition of "outcome." It may go far beyond the physical experience, such as the remission of a disease. A positive outcome may mean that by living a positive, enjoyable life, by enjoying the "process," you achieve an outcome of spiritual peace even though the physical outcome is death. I believe that and I also believe that a positive outcome can be defined as personal growth, in which people so transcend their pain that they eventually view the pain as a blessing because of the growth it brought.

Come to your own understanding of the motivational power of belief in your life. A positive outcome can be pursued while recognizing the beauty and fulfillment of the process of living. See the small, daily tasks of life for the enjoyment and reward they can bring.

> Look to this day
> for it is the very life of Life.
> In its brief course lie all
> the verities and realities
> of your existence.
> For yesterday is but a dream and tomorrow is only a vision.
> But today well-lived makes
> every yesterday a dream of Happiness
> and every tomorrow a vision of Hope.
> Look well, therefore, to this day
> It is the life of Life!
>
> Sanskrit

Summary

* Motivation is both a vital energy for carrying out healthy behaviors and a limitless fuel to keep the flame of hope burning.

* Hopelessness is a major obstacle to motivation, and it must be countered by positive self-talk and a positive self-image.

* You will be motivated by those things in life that you value most.

* You will be motivated to change behaviors if you have input into the decisions that affect you.

* You must set your own goals for managing your disease, using information and advice from trusted medical and personal advisors.

* Set goals in small achievable steps so that success can build on success.

* Choose rewards for yourself and give them often to motivate you to achieve further success.

* You can benefit from positive reinforcement in two ways: train your internal coach to give you regular positive comments, and go out of your way to make positive comments about other people.

* "Pokers are the people, places, and experiences in life that renew and energize us. Define your "pokers" and make use of them to keep yourself "up."

* Belief in a positive outcome is a powerful motivator for healthy behaviors.

* Expectations become self-fulfilling prophecy.

* Visualizing yourself looking healthy now and in the future will increase your positive belief.

* You must visualize *and* believe in your chosen outcome.

* Positive outcome does not necessarily mean a completely healthy future or remission or a cure for your disease. Enjoying the process of life will lead to a healthy outlook and spiritual growth, in whatever fashion you define it.

Reflection Questions

1. Reflect on what a "fulfilling life" means to you. This is the foundation for your motivation. It is what you hope for, what you live for. Close your eyes and see yourself participating in this happy, healthy, fulfilling life. Be specific in your vision.

What do you look like?

Where are you?

What are you doing?

Who is with you?

How do you feel?

What changes do you need to make to enable that vision to come true?

List three steps you can take right now that will lead you toward your fulfilling life. Consider these "steps" to be your goals.

2. Identify any hopelessness that you feel about your ability to achieve your goals. Describe this feeling in your own words:

Choose a trusted counselor or friend to discuss this feeling with, and *do* it.

3. Follow the advice in this chapter for setting goals. If you experience any difficulty, ask a friend or member of your medical team to assist you.

Chapter 4

Adapting To Life's Challenges

Adaptability may be one of the most important qualities of a healthy life. The circumstances of life are changing continually. Either we adapt to fit these changing circumstances or our well-being suffers. As I look back over a variety of challenging circumstances in my life I feel that one of my most helpful assets is the ability to adapt.

> Daddy died when I was nine years old. When my Brownie troop held its first father-daughter banquet I could have chosen not to attend. Instead I invited Daddy's best friend to be my escort. It became a fun tradition which he and I enjoyed all the years I was in scouting. I miss my father to this day, but I did adapt to life without him.

When I was ten years old I got diabetes. Living well with my diabetes has been a continuing exercise in adaptability. As a ten-year-old I went to slumber parties and brought all my equipment with me so I could do my testing and give my shots. Likewise, I went on Girl Scout campouts, played in the marching band, and participated in sports. Having diabetes just meant I had to think through a few more situations than the other kids—I had to adapt.

My need for adaptability will continue to be challenged throughout my life. Once I flew to a meeting and the airline confirmed twice that the flight was a meal flight. Once aboard the plane, however, I was told there was no food. That's a potentially serious situation for a person with insulin-dependent diabetes who isn't prepared to adapt. I adapted to the situation by eating food I had brought with me.

Personality tests indicate that adaptability is an inherent quality. Some people are by nature highly adaptable, while others find it very difficult to adapt. Among the most humane people in medicine are those who accept individual differences in their patients' ability to adapt. But those same wise health professionals know that everyone, except for the seriously mentally ill, can choose to improve their ability to adapt. Once an individual has made the choice to improve, he or she can learn skills and find the necessary support to make healthy adaptations to the changing circumstances of life.

Many life events require adaptation

Adaptation is not a skill reserved just for living well with a disease. It is a necessary part of every healthy life. Just think of all the times people *have* to adapt!

* When the fourth person shows up for dinner and there are three chicken breasts. (Your menu changes to stir fry chicken!)

* When the projector bulb burns out in the middle of a slide presentation. (You quickly learn to graphically describe visuals.)

* Getting laid off from a job. (Teaches you creativity as you live more simply.)

* Spraining the thumb on your writing hand when you have a paper due tomorrow. (Typing is slow without your thumb, but you make it.)

That's life. You adapt to its changing circumstances because you must. To do otherwise would mean giving up and missing out on what life has to offer to her survivors. One of the important qualities that makes people survivors is their ability to adapt. Many people must adapt to a challenge to their health — it is one of the most crucial adaptations anyone can make.

Eventually we all are confronted with the challenge of coping with physical limitation, whether it be from disease, illness, injury, or simply aging. Each of us must make our own separate peace with this issue. People with a disease or injury face this challenge earlier in their lives. People who are basically free of disease all their lives meet the issue of physical limitation when they reach an age at which their body systems are simply slowing down.

The following describes a beautiful attitude with which to meet physical limitation. If you can hold and adopt this attitude, then your limitation will truly be confined to the physical.

> I like spring, but it is too young. I like summer, but it is too proud. So I like best of all autumn; because its leaves are a little yellow, its tone mellower, it colors richer. And it is tinged a little with sorrow. Its golden richness speaks not of the innocence of spring, nor of the power of summer, but of the mellowness and kindly wisdom of approaching age. It knows the limitations of life and is content.
>
> Lin Yutang

One of my family's most treasured friends lived to be 97 years old. Throughout the wonderful years that we knew Bob, we were continually inspired by his healthy approach to life and living. It delights me to remember that he bowled on a league until he was 96! Over the years we bowled with him we did see a gradual decline in his "approach" to the bowling alley. But his approach to life never waivered. He was very pragmatic about his declining physical state. Only occasionally would he mention that he noticed about every five years that he wasn't quite able to do what he had five years earlier. Most of the time Bob talked of the future. He was forward-thinking, active, and full of the life around him. Although he outlived two wives and spent his last years alone, he never seemed lonely. We invited Bob to our home frequently; not because we felt sorry for him, but because we thoroughly enjoyed him as a stimulating, inspiring friend. Because he adapted to his challenges with such peace, strength, and humor, I regard him as one of my most important role models.

Many people face adaptation to physical limitation much earlier in their lives. The person who becomes near-sighted gets glasses. This common and relatively minor adaptation allows him or her to see well again and continue enjoying a visually healthy life.

People with allergies or asthma adapt to their challenge by avoiding the food or other source of their allergic reaction. Some people require medication or even as great an adaptation as a move to another part of the country.

People with diabetes must make adaptations in their entire lifestyle. To successfully adapt to the disease's requirements they must eat according to a prescribed meal plan and time schedule. Some need to take pills or daily injections of insulin. Most people with diabetes are instructed to do daily finger stick blood tests to determine if their blood sugar is within a healthy range. Daily exercise and ongoing stress management are also necessary if one is to live well with diabetes.

People recovering from a heart attack or heart surgery must adapt their work schedule, exercise and activity, meals, and stress management. Medications and medical equipment may also become a necessary part of a healthy life.

Each health challenge presents its own demands, each of which requires *adaptation*.

Obviously, adaptation is not always as easy as getting a pair of glasses and wearing them. Some health challenges are very complex. The medical aspects of a healthy adaptation to one's disease require a highly skilled and committed team of health care providers to give advice on the physical requirements posed by each health challenge. Each of you reading this book must take the responsibility to find a medical resource to advise you on how to live well with your health challenge by making wise and healthy adaptations. This book does not deal with the medical aspects of diseases. It looks at the human side of adapting one's life to accomodate the requirements of a disease while still pursuing one's hopes and dreams for a happy, fulfilling life.

Adapt rather than accept

An interesting study was done some years ago using infants. A cold, metal sheet was laid next to the infants in a bassinet. Some of the babies turned away from the cold as soon as they felt it. Other babies simply lay there and cried.

The adaptability and spirit of the first group of babies is similar to the spirit found in a group called the Candlelighters. They are a group of parents whose children have cancer. They get together to offer support to themselves and others. They have chosen to light a candle instead of cursing the darkness.

Acceptance of one's disease or the limitations it imposes can be negative if it leads to resignation or giving up hope. Acceptance is negative if it stops people unnecessarily from doing what they want to do.

Norman Cousins is an excellent role model of health and well-being. In his tremendous book, *Anatomy of an Illness*, Cousins tells his true story of a remarkable recovery from a very serious disease. He was diagnosed with a serious collagen disease and told that he had only a 1 in 500 chance for recovery. Instead of giving up and waiting to die, he got busy with his own recovery.

Cousins was aware of the negative impact stress has on the body. He believed that stress had triggered his disease. So, he reasoned, if stress does negative things to the body, why can't the opposite emotions have a positive impact? If stress kills, why can't love, self-confidence, the will to live, faith, and laughter heal? Cousins tested his theory in part by viewing Marx Brothers movies and Candid Camera Classics. He found that a ten-minute belly laugh gave him two hours of pain-free sleep. And, after each episode of laughter, the sedimentation rate of his blood dropped. (This was the chemical indicator of his disease.) The drop was small, but it held and was cumulative. Cousins laughed himself to a total recovery.

Norman Cousins refused to blindly accept a negative prognosis. If he had chosen acceptance rather than adaptation, he would have resigned himself to progressive paralysis and death. Instead, he chose to look for an answer to his problem. His lack of acceptance led to his eventual recovery.

The opposite of acceptance is denial. And just as there are both healthy and unhealthy forms of acceptance, there are also healthy and unhealthy forms of denial. Cousins found a healthy way to deny his prognosis. Sometimes it is difficult to distinguish between a healthy and an unhealthy denial. Parents often ignore a child's vague complaint of a "tummy ache," hoping to discourage the use of illness as an attention-getter or a responsibility-avoider. However, when should you pay attention to a tummy ache? A friend of mine who is a pediatrician missed her son's appendicitis with the "oh-you'll-be-just-fine" approach!

Denial is unhealthy when it leads to unhealthy consequences. Denial of disease can lead to a worsening of the disease if the individual doesn't take medication and follow other healthy behaviors necessary to control it. It's hard to deny health challenges that have obvious consequences, such as the amputation of a limb. But many diseases are invisible, causing only internal effects and possibly vague physical symptoms. Hypertension (high blood pressure) is called the silent killer because it causes few if any symptoms. Denying it can be deadly. Likewise, a woman who detects a breast lump but does not have it checked is denying its possible threat at great risk to her future well-being.

Diabetes is another insidious killer and crippler which can be denied for years with little negative consequence. Then, after years of high blood sugars people can suffer devastating consequences such as blindness and kidney failure. The irony is that some people feel that by taking care of their disease they are giving in to it and allowing it to take control of their life. Healthy people realize that by learning how to take care of their disease and then following the required healthy behaviors they are taking control not only of their disease but of their life.

Seek a healthy balance between denial and acceptance. Each of us must find our own level of comfort and balance. If you're unclear about the health or "illth" of your denial, talk it over with a trusted advisor such as your physician.

Adaptability requires practicality

A practical and realistic attitude about one's disease is the starting point from which to discover healthy adaptations to it.

> I heard of a man whose hand had been seriously burned when he was a child. Because he did not receive the necessary plastic surgery, his hand is now permanently partially closed. Anyone who has tried getting along with just one hand for any length of time knows what a problem that is. That is not how this man approached his challenge, however. He stated his wonderfully practical approach as follows: "Problems by definition can be solved. My hand is not a problem to me. It is a fact of life. I just do as much as I can with it and do the rest with my other hand."

Try taking this man's approach: Think of your disease as he does his partially closed hand. Adapt to the challenge, not the problem. Do as much as you can with your disease, and do the rest with your "other hand," which is everything not affected by your disease.

Dr. William Menninger of the famed Menninger Foundation and Clinic composed a list he called, "Criteria for Emotional Maturity." The first criterion on the list is: "The ability to deal constructively with reality." That is an excellent definition of adaptability.

Dealing constructively with reality means avoiding the pitfall of "If only . . ." People who fall into this pit spend their whole life saying, "If only things were different, then I would be happy." The thought can take many forms: If only I were married (or single); If only I had a child (or some child-free time to myself); If only I had a new house, a new job, a new wardrobe, a different spouse, a disease-free body. If only (fill in the blank), then my life would be good.

"If only" is not reality. The people who successfully avoid this pitfall are those who make the best of any situation in which they find themselves. They successfully adapt their lifestyle to fit their income. They get busy finding things to like about their job, their spouse, and their home instead of constantly complaining. They look beyond the negative to find the positive. They continue to find fulfillment in life even after they get a disease.

> "We have to take reality as it comes to us: there is no good jabbering about what it ought to be like or what we should have expected it to be like."
>
> C.S. Lewis

Disease is a detour, not a destination

Disease or disability does not have to be a destination or an end point in one's life. Death is surely an end point, but to resign oneself to death because a disease or disability has entered one's life is to deny life itself. This book addresses living well with health challenges that are chronic in nature;

that is, they occur over a long period of time. That generally means that an individual who gets a chronic disease lives with it for months or years. The disease is not a destination in itself. Life does not end with the disease, but because it is chronic the disease becomes part of one's life. Because most diseases present challenges in life and living, they do need to be viewed realisticaly as detours.

Viewing disease or disability as a detour means that your goal for a fulfilling life remains the same, but the path leading to that goal has been blocked. In order to adapt, you must find an alternate route to reach that goal. *Study* is essential if you are going to be able to read the road map of life and successfully find a way around your roadblock. *Study* your disease and learn all that is required for you to live well with it. *Study* healthy living in general and as much as possible integrate the requirements of your disease with the recommendations of healthy living. *Study* yourself. It is essential that you understand your real goal for life.

I have heard numerous people express the opinion that a benefit they have derived from having a disease is the clarity it brought in defining what's *really* important in life. Being confronted by a disease brings people face-to-face with their mortality. Sometimes it is only after this confrontation that people make delightful discoveries like:

* How sweet the spring air smells after a rain

* The exquisite beauty of each unique snowflake

* The priceless melody in a child's laugh

* The profound satisfaction in loving and being loved

This confrontation can also help people discern what is only superficially important and what is really important in helping them to reach their life's goal. I observed a blind friend of mine as she overcame the obstacle of blindness to reach her life's goal of being a good mother.

My friend lost her sight when her daughter was in first

grade. Among her greatest struggles with her blindness was the feeling that it diminished her as a mother. This feeling of sadness and loss caused her to closely examine her role as a mother.

She realized that she had held the opinion that "a good mother develops her child's curiosity and intelligence through reading." Beginning to view her blindness as a detour, she realized that she could still encourage her daughter's reading without doing the reading herself. My friend and her daughter enjoyed many hours cuddling on the sofa as they listened to cassette tapes of great children's literature.

Sometimes it takes extraordinary determination to adapt to one's challenge. One of my heroes demonstrated this determination in adapting to life with one arm.

Dick is a physician and father of four. He has had only one arm since he was 11 months old, when he stuck his arm in his mother's washing machine. Every step along the path of his life required adaptation: learning to tie his shoes, playing baseball, and, of course, the many challenges he met in medical school.

Family support was crucial to Dick's adaptability. His parents insisted that he learn to tie his shoes like the other five-year-olds. His father spent many hours teaching him how to catch a baseball, quickly get the glove off and throw the ball. Dick lettered in high school baseball.

By the time Dick entered medical school he truly viewed his challenge as only a detour. During the surgical rotation he tied his surgical mask with one hand and found every other alternative route necessary to take him to the goals he set for himself.

Learn by observing others

"Through appreciation we make the excellence in others our own property."

Voltaire

Besides receiving inspiration from the stories of brave people who have adapted to their health challenge, you can also learn helpful and practical techniques for adapting to your own challenge.

People with arthritis can find that mobility problems need not make them immobile. By allowing extra time, planning a route that does not present obstacles such as steep stairs, and asking for the support of helpful friends and relatives, the challenge to adapt can be met.

People with digestive disorders can enjoy restaurant eating by finding restaurants that serve appropriate food or are willing to prepare food as the customer requires.

It would be impossible to describe all the adaptations required of individuals with a chronic health challenge. You need to study and learn to adapt to your own challenges, and a good way to start is by observing how others with your disease or disability adapt to their challenges. To find those individuals, look in your phone book under the disease or disability you have. If there is a local branch of a national organization like the American Cancer Society, Arthritis Foundation, Diabetes Association, Heart Association, or other group, call them. Find out what services they provide. If they hold educational meetings or support groups, attend them. Meet people who are adapting successfully to your health challenge and learn how they do it. If there is no such group in your community, ask at the public library for the address of the national headquarters for your disease. Write and ask them to send helpful information about living with the disease and about the services they provide. Find out what it would take to set up a local branch in your community.

After studying and observing others, you will be ready to

apply what you have learned. Try different techniques, and if they help you, keep at it. *Evaluate.* If a particular adaptation is not helpful, then keep studying and observing until you find techniques that do help you adapt successfully.

Nothing in this book is an absolute. Everything must be studied, observed, applied, and evaluated by *you.* That's how to learn to adapt. It is a continuing process because life is ever-changing. The challenges arise. The detours change. Even the goals evolve over time. The only healthy answer is to be able to continually adapt to maintain your well-being and your progress toward your goal of a fulfilling life.

Adaptability provides hope that you will reach your destination. And, at its best, it helps you enjoy the journey.

Summary

* Adaptability is one of the most helpful assets a person can have, because life's circumstances are always changing. Some people naturally adapt to major changes better than others, but everyone can learn to improve his or her ability to adapt in order to live well with a chronic disease.

* Everyone faces the challenge of physical limitations—it's called aging. Just as aging requires a positive yet realistic approach to living life to its fullest, so does a chronic disease require a positive determination to adapt and do as much as possible with what is left in life.

* A highly skilled and committed team of health care providers can be the key to successful adaptation for an individual with a chronic disease.

* There is a healthy way of denying one's disease as well as an unhealthy way. Denial is unhealthy when it leads to a worsening of one's disease and/or detracts from one's ability to live well. Denial is healthy when it motivates an individual to do everything possible to live fully and take control of one's disease.

* Successful adapters are busy finding things to like about every part of life. They take a practical approach to doing as much as they can with whatever limitations they have been handed in life.

* Disease is a detour, not a destination.

* Learn from others who have successfully adapted to life with the disease you have. Then, enjoy your journey to the destination you have mapped out for your life.

Reflection Questions

1. Make a list of the requirements placed on you by your disease.

   Medications:

   Therapy:

   Diet:

   Exercise:

   Changes in lifestyle:

   Other:

2. Write a description of how you work these requirements into a happy, fulfilling life. When you have done that, you have adapted!

You and Stress: Who is in Control?

The phone never stops ringing at work. There are more orders than you can possibly process. Your manager is pushing you to keep up. You work overtime. As soon as you walk in the door at home your spouse begins to complain about your being late. You open your mail and learn that your parents plan to visit you and stay for three weeks. Your muscles tighten. You are experiencing

STRESS.

Life is going relatively smoothly for you. You enjoy your work. Your family life is fulfilling. You have several hobbies you enjoy. Your carefuly planned investments are beginning to show the promise of a comfortable retirement. Then, you visit your physician for a routine examination. You are told that you have a chronic, incurable disease. The message is clear. It can't be fixed. It might be controllable. It will change the way you live. Your eyes fill with tears as you respond to

STRESS.

In the process of living, stress is inevitable. It is suggested that the absence of stress occurs only at death. So, we must learn how to live successfully with the stresses of life. If you can do that, then *you* are in control. Stress becomes a form of energy, an important force that enables you to be a creative, productive, exciting person. If you cannot learn how to live successfully with life's stresses, then stress becomes the controlling force in your life. It may dissipate your energy, leaving you frustrated and unhappy, or it may even crush your spirit and leave you totally unable to function.

The stress of a disease

Control is central to successful stress management. Even though you could not control getting a disease, you have a great deal of control over how much stress it will cause you. Concepts discussed in the chapters on self-image and adaptability will have a major impact on how much control you have over stress. If you can maintain a positive self-image and adapt successfully to the ongoing requirements of your disease, then the disease will not be an overwhelming source of stress to you.

Positive self-talk (described in the self-image chapter) is an important stress management technique. It addresses one of the most basic observations made by stress management experts:

Stress is not an event.
It is our perception of the event.

Dr. George E. Vaillant, Raymond Sobel Proffessor of Psychiatry, Dartmouth Medical School and Director of the Study of Adult Development, Dartmouth Medical School and Harvard University Health Services, illustrates this concept by describing a group of people on a roller coaster, having fun and even looking relaxed after the ride. He finds such rides to be stressful. It is the same event, but some find it fun while others feel it is stressful. The difference is in the way the event is viewed, or perceived, by each individual. A disease is an event in life. How it is perceived determines how much stress it causes in one's life.

When Georgia got diabetes, she was shocked and sad. She loved rich desserts and was sad to think she must now give them up. For awhile she was mostly sad as she counted ler losses. Then, she grew dissatisfied with all the sadness in her life and, after talking with her medical team and several close friends, she began to practice this technique of choosing positive thoughts instead of the negative, sad thoughts. Following is an example of how she has taught herself to choose positive thoughts.

When Georgia begins to feel sad because she can't eat a rich dessert, she goes through this type of thought process: "Oh, how I miss pecan pie! Well, the truth is I simply can't eat it anymore because I have diabetes. Actually, no one should eat it. It has an enormous number of calories— nearly 800. That's more than half the number of calories I need in a whole day. Those calories, though, are not nutritious, vitamin, mineral and fiber-filled calories. They are sugary, fatty, empty calories. I am much better off with my new lifestyle of healthy, nutritious eating.

"There are consequences for nearly everything we do. The consequences of eating pecan pie include the risk of gaining weight, having high blood sugars and contributing to the artery-clogging effect of eating saturated fat. A few moments of sweet taste are not worth those risks. Now, instead of sitting here thinking about pie, what can I do that would be fun? I think I'll call Anne and see if she'd like to walk around the lake. It will be nice to see Anne, to see how the trees are blooming and a walk will be invigorating and healthy!

"I know that I could make myself miserable by sitting here contemplating my losses. I choose not to do that. I will instead do something enjoyable and healthy. I am a strong and intelligent person. I have just made a healthy, wise choice."

Georgia has learned that thoughts create feelings. Sad thoughts make her feel sad. She chooses not to feel sad. The positive thoughts she gives herself create just the feelings she wants.

Dr. Vaillant describes altered perceptions and other successful stress management techniques as "ingenious adaptation to stress." One conclusion he draws from his research is that, "Stress does not kill us so much as ingenious adaptation to stress facilitates (helps) our survival." Make an ingenious adaptation to your disease by giving yourself positive messages to replace the negative ones. Don't say, "Poor me, I have a disease. My life is all but over." Instead, say, "I have a real challenge ahead of me, but it isn't the end of the world. I'll learn what I can and face this as well as I can with dignity and strength." It isn't easy. You will need all the support you can muster. Techniques and resources for gaining that support will be discussed in later chapters.

If you feel that you are not making progress in managing the stress of your disease, then please, seek counseling. That is a very wise step toward well-being, because counselors are excellent teachers of ingenious adaptations to stress. The following feelings and situations are signs of depression. One or more of them may be your signal to seek professional support.

Feelings of helplessness and hopelessness, feeling trapped.
Sad feelings and crying without knowing why or for very minor reasons.
Feeling confused and unable to make decisions.
Finding it difficult to function in daily routines.

Withdrawal from others . . . wanting to be left alone.
Dependence on chemicals such as sleeping pills,
tranquilizers, or alcohol to keep you going.
Feeling worthless.
Caught up in feelings of resentment or self-pity.

From Lutheran Social Services

The diagnosis of a disease can cause a great deal of initial
stress. However, stress related to your disease can recur
throughout your life. You will never master your disease any
more than you will ever master life. Living well with your
disease means that you learn continually how to cope with it
and the stress it causes.

Because I was a child when I was diagnosed with diabetes, it
was my mother who had most of the stress to manage.
Because she did that so beautifully, I managed very well.
When I got into my teens I was assuming more of the
care-taking responsibility, and I was also experiencing more
of the stress.

When I was 17 I became eligible for a travel/study program
through my high school. But when I reviewed the program's
requirements, I read that "Diabetics and epileptics need not
apply." I was furious! That was *SO* unfair. Then, I was asked by
the selection committee to serve as a member of that group in
choosing a student for the program. "Why, they've taken a
disappointment and turned it into an honor," my mother
quickly pointed out to me. She convinced me of that. My new
"perception" alleviated my stress.

When I was thinking of getting married I was experiencing
stress as I thought of all the terrible things diabetes could do
to me and what that would mean for a husband. Before
becoming engaged I went to see my physician. I wanted him
to give me a definitive answer. I wanted to hear either "Do not
get married, because there is always the possibility that you
won't do well," or "Go ahead and get married, because I know
you are going to do well . . . and live happily ever after." In a

very caring way, my wonderful physician talked sense to me. He told me that absolutely no one knows what the future will bring. Today's decisions are made without any guarantees about tomorrow. I came to the realization that:

A health challenge does not make life any more uncertain. It simply makes us aware of the uncertainty of life.

Dale and I married. Less than a year later a classmate of his had a double mastectomy. Life is uncertain. And so precious.

Because I value motherhood so highly, I have experienced some of my most powerful and poignant struggles with diabetes as I have perceived it threatening that role. I nursed my baby. While I nursed, my blood sugars would often get low as my body used up calories for milk production. One night I awakened to John's fiercely hungry cry. As I jumped out of bed I realized that my blood sugar was low. Because the maternal instinct to tend to my baby was so strong, I seriously considered nursing him first, then eating later. However, as I walked toward his bedroom I realized that I was *quite* hypoglycemic, so I quickly detoured downstairs for a quick glass of juice. When I got to John's bedroom I found my husband, holding our squalling bit of humanity, trying to comfort him. Dale had figured that I needed to boost my blood sugar, so as he gently rocked John he said to him, "Sometimes Mom has to eat first."

That very nearly broke my heart. Moms don't do *anything* first, or so my culture has taught me. That was a very sad moment in my life. However, by the clear light of dawn I was able to talk sense to myself and return some balance to my perception of the situation. I reminded myself that when my blood sugar is low I am very vulnerable emotionally and thus would perceive the situation as being far more dire than it actually was. Then I sort of took myself by the shoulders and said, "That's right. Sometimes, *in order* to be a good mother you DO have to eat first, but you're still a good Mom." I sincerely felt the issue to be settled, the stress resolved. Again, it is the perception of the event that creates or removes stress.

Your disease must likewise be taken into account as you confront every major life event. Consider positive self-talk as your most important ally. It can take you from anger to understanding, from sadness to a tolerable frustration, and even, from doubt to hope.

Successful management of day-to-day stress is important to everyone who wishes to live a healthy, happy life. And successful stress management is even more important for people who have a disease. Unmanaged stress can make an existing disease worse. Unhealthy ways of coping with stress, such as smoking, drinking, and eating, can worsen one's disease. The rest of this chapter will help you define the daily stresses in your life and will discuss ways to control how much stress they cause you.

The stress of life

Just as disease-related stress can recur thoughout one's life, so is the stress of life an ongoing fact. Healthy people learn to cope with routine stress because they realize that no one masters life. Just when parents feel they have mastered infant care, the infant turns into a toddler . . . Happily married people have not mastered marriage. They have learned to continually nourish, nurture, and develop their relationship so that they can cope with the inevitable challenges in any marriage. Coping is not simply a nice little life skill to help life go more smoothly. It is absolutely essential to anyone who wishes to live a healthy life.

Whether it is family life, work life, social life, or one's personal life, no one ever reaches a point where they are no longer confronted with challenges. (Think about this: If you suddenly found yourself with no challenges, that in itself would be a major challenge, because you would need to find some meaningful direction for your life.) Stress produced by life's challenges is not only inevitable, it is essential for fulfillment. A challenge can be a positive form of stress or a negative form of stress, depending on how you perceive it and cope with it. A violin provides an excellent analogy of the importance of stress in one's life. If violin strings have no stress (tension) then the violin can produce no music. But you know what happens when too much stress is applied to the violin's strings: They snap. You need to become a "coper" so that YOU don't snap, but rather, enjoy the symphony of life!

Know your stress signals

How can you tell when the stress in your life has gotten out of hand? What are the signals that alert you? Some common signals include: headache, short temper, fatigue, feeling anxious, diarrhea, aching muscles, neck soreness, and jaw pain. You may experience a flare up of the symptoms of your disease. My diabetes is very reactive to stress. I have high blood sugars and ketones (signs of an acid imbalance) when I am under too much stress.

Know yourself. People experience stress very differently. Some people always experience headaches; some people never do. For some people the first clue of excessive stress is an increase in a behavior they use to cope with stress. Thus, one person's signal may be an increase in drinking. Another may have a tendency to snack constantly. Once you become aware of your stress signal, figure out what is causing it.

Know the cause of your stress

Whenever possible, trace your stress signal to its source. ("This headache began just after the board meeting when it was announced that sales quotas would be looked at more closely than ever.") Sometimes the source of your stress will be quite obvious to you. Below is a partial list of some common sources of stress. Do you see yours listed?

* Deadlines; feeling time pressure
* Having too much to do and not enough time or help to get it done.
* Having to report to too many people: boss, spouse, children,

parents; being pulled in too many directions.
* Feeling out of control of your life.
* Sense of being behind: your friends make more money, have nicer homes, accomplish more, get better promotions, or just seem to have a better life than you do.
* Personal dissatisfaction: You should lose (or gain) weight but can't, you know you shouldn't smoke but can't quit, you should have reached a higher educational level but haven't, you should have married someone else, you should quit your job but don't want to take the risk, etc. (The *"shoulds"* are very powerful, negative stressors.)
* Your disease and fears for the future are frustrating your efforts to make changes in your present lifestyle.
* Big decisions: Career? Marriage? Children? Move? Change jobs? Retire?

List as many other sources of stress as you perceive in your life. You may list sources that are highly stressful as well as those that are only small irritations. Some stress experts believe that chronic small irritations are ultimately more stressful and take a greater toll than occasional major stress.

Control the controllable

Once you have determined the source of your stress, decide if it can be removed. It it can be, remove the stress. Control what you can. You may realize that you've worked too many hours on a particular project. You may remove the stress by stopping work to relax, or by working on something less stressful for awhile, or by quitting a job that is just too stressful.

Your stress may be caused by anger toward someone. You may remove this stress by confronting the conflict you are having with another person and resolving it. You may be dreading making a phone call. Make the call. Get it done. Remove the stress.

There are times when you may experience what is called "episodic" stress, when for a brief time there is an almost unavoidable stress (tax time, house guests), but that you know will end. You can cope with this type of stress simply by reminding yourself often that it *will* end. This will give you more of a feeling of control over the situation. *Control* is the central issue with stress management.

Look over the list of sources of stress. Make your own list of the sources of stress in your life. Place a "C" in front of those you feel you can control, and make a commitment to do just that at every opportunity.

Cope with the stress you cannot control

Once you have controlled as much stress as possible, you can learn to cope with the rest. The following suggestions are practical methods for coping with stress. Learn about and experiment with each coping method to find specific methods that work for you in two different ways:

1) To actively alleviate stress during the time you are experiencing your stress signals or are under extreme temporary stress, so that you avoid negative coping behaviors; and

2) To use as a preventive measure, by practicing one or more of the coping methods on a daily or several times weekly basis, so that your stress is not allowed to build up to a harmful level.

Altered perception through self-talk

Thoughts create feelings. To relieve stressful feelings, change your thoughts. When my husband was working hard to get his new business going, he came home one day looking extremely tired. He said to me, "I'll bet the phone rang 200 times today!" Then, before I could respond, he grinned and said, "Business is good!"

Since work-related stress is so common, let me share one of my favorite perspectives on the subject:

Benefits of Trouble
The Rev. John Wesley Ford

"Be thankful for the troubles of your job. They provide about half your income, because if it were not for the things that go wrong, the difficult people you have to deal with, and the problems and unpleasantness of your working day, someone could be found to handle your job for half of what you are being paid.

> "It takes intelligence, resourcefulness, patience, tact, and courage to meet the troubles of any job. That is why you hold your present job. If all of us would start to look for more troubles and learn to handle them cheerfully and with good judgment as opportunities rather than irritation, we would find ourselves getting ahead at a surprising rate, for it is a fact that there are plenty of big jobs waiting for those who aren't afraid of the troubles connected with them."

Exercise

Choose a physical activity suitable to your specific needs *and* one you enjoy. That adds *fun*, which is another great stress reducer!

For those who can, a good, brisk, arm-swinging walk is one of the best exercises. Vigorous exercise should be cleared with your doctor. (Exercise should reduce stress, not create it!)

Reinforce your enjoyment by inviting a friend to join you. You'll be more likely to exercise regularly, and you'll also be promoting your friend's health.

Laughter

> "The mind ought sometimes to be amused, that it may the better return to thought, and to itself."

> Phaedrus (5th century BC)

Make your own list of the sources of laughter in your life, such as funny movies, friends, books, games, and events.

Be aware of the humor in day-to-day living. Be open to and ready for laughter. (Enjoy the sign you may see in a cafeteria: "Shoes required to eat in cafeteria," and ask your lunch companion, "I wonder where socks have to eat")

Especially be open to laughing at yourself. Don't take life or yourself too seriously.

Remember:

> "A merry heart doeth good like a medicine, but a broken spirit drieth the bones."
>
> Proverbs 17:22

Vacation

Take a real vacation—completely cut off from your daily routine—on a regular basis.

Everyone needs to renew, recharge, and relax.

Music

Choose your favorite music and spend time with it as you would spend time with a favorite friend.

> "Life can't be all bad when for ten dollars you can buy all the Beethoven sonatas and listen to them for ten years."
>
> William F. Buckley, Jr.

> "Bach opens a vista to the universe. After experiencing him people feel there is meaning to life after all."
>
> Helmut Walcha

Some people choose soothing music when they want to relax, and some choose rousing music when they want to be inspired and stimulated. Music can both relax and energize!

Relaxation Techniques

Find a quiet place where you are comfortable and can be undisturbed for 20 minutes. Sit awhile with your eyes closed.

Get a picture in your mind of a huge gunny sack and, one by one, drop all of your worries and burdens into it. Begin a progressive muscle relaxation exercise, starting with your scalp and facial muscles. Alternately tighten each muscle group and then relax it. Go to the next muscle group and continue this technique of flexing for several seconds, then releasing and relaxing the muscles, group by group, until you reach your toes.

You may want to do progressive relaxation to relaxing music of your choice. Some people record their own voice giving them the instructions to tighten and relax the specific muscle groups.

For a quick relaxer, try deep breathing. Slowly take in a deep breath. Breathe in as much air as you can possibly hold. Then, slowly let all the air out. When I do this I tell myself on the inhale that I am breathing in energy. On the exhale I tell myself that I am expelling all my stress. It works!

Visualization

Once you are in a relaxed state, you are ready to experience further relaxation through visualization. To do this, remember a time and place where you felt relaxed and happy. Close your eyes. "See" yourself relaxed and happy at your chosen location. Now, remember it with all your senses. What do you see, hear, feel, smell, taste? Here's an example using my favorite visualization:

> I see myself sitting next to a fire on a beach. I am smiling and I look peaceful. I hear the crackling of the wood as it burns. I also hear the waves lapping into shore. I feel the heat from the fire. I also feel the cool, silkiness of the sand as I run my toes and fingers through it. I smell the smoke of the fire and the distinct but pleasant smell of the river. I am at peace. I am relaxed.

Have mental pictures that are very soothing and appealing. Visit them often as if you were taking a brief vacation. Keep pictures of your favorite place on your desk or countertop to remind you to take that mini-vacation.

location for relaxation:

choice of background music:

favorite visualization

I see . . .

I hear . . .

I smell . . .

I feel . . .

I taste . . .

I am relaxed.

Besides visualizing, keep dreaming. In the Self-Image chapter Dr. Frederick Engstrom described how important day-dreams are. Dreaming is also important in day-to-day coping. It is dreams which lift us above our troubles and give us hope. As Langston Hughes expresses it:

Hold fast to dreams
For if Dreams die
Life is a broken-winged bird
That cannot fly.

Hold fast to dreams
For when dreams go
Life is a barren field
Frozen with snow.

Meditation and Prayer

Find a quiet environment where you will be undisturbed and feel that you have privacy. Relax yourself by the progressive technique. Compose a prayer or meditation to suit your personal needs and beliefs. Meditation can also be a non-religious experience in which you reflect on all the good in your world and receive both peace and inspiration. You may choose to reflect on the words of a good book, the inspiring life of a friend or world leader, or the serenity found in nature.

Here is an interesting thought regarding religion and stress:

> "Religious faith is not a storm cellar to which men and women can flee for refuge from the storms of life. It is, instead, an inner spiritual strength that enables them to face those storms with hope and serenity. Religious faith has the miraculous power to lift ordinary human beings to greatness in seasons of stress. Religious faith is to be found in the promises of God."

> Sen. Sam J. Ervin, Jr.

The following is a translation of a Japanese variation of the 23rd Psalm:

> The Lord is my pace-setter; I shall not rush.
> He makes me stop and rest for quiet intervals;
> He provides me with images of stillness
> which restore my serenity.
> He leads me in the ways of efficiency through
> calmness of mind,
> And His guidance is my peace.
> Even though I have a great many things
> to accomplish each day,
> I will not fret, for His presence is here.
> His timelessness, His all-importance, will
> keep me in balance.
> He prepares refreshment and renewal in
> the midst of my activity,

By annointing my mind with His oils of tranquility.
My cup of joyous energy overflows.
Surely harmony and effectiveness shall be
the fruit of my hours,
For I shall walk in the pace of my Lord
and dwell in His house forever.

Toki Miyashina

(Reproduced by kind permission of The Saint Andrew Press, Edinburgh, Scotland.)

Support Network

Select a friend who has experienced the type of stress you are experiencing — preferably one who has successfully overcome it. Talk about it. Express your feelings. Telling a trusted friend what's bothering you helps to clarify your thoughts. And you may find a resolution for the stress as you listen to yourself. If no one in your support system seems to understand you, do not hesitate to get professional counseling.

Be part of someone else's support network. Hans Selye, physician and noted stress management expert, considered this to be one of the most important ways to manage stress. He called it "altruistic egotism." When we help others, we help ourselves. There are many charitable organizations and agencies in need of your help. Perhaps the most gratifying giving is that which is done in person. Find someone you can visit, assist, cheer up, or help in any way.

One of our son's friends broke his leg in a hockey game. He had to be in traction in the hospital for more than two weeks. It was a tough time for an 11-year-old boy and his family. Instinctively, we reached out to this family, and as we did, we felt our own continued healing. Below is an excerpt from the letter I wrote our young friend when he left the hospital:

"You will never be the same person because of your broken leg. You are a better, stronger, wiser person. You may not be aware of that yet. But, someday you will hear of a little boy who has broken his leg (playing hockey, skiing, or in a car accident) and is hospitalized in traction. Your heart will tell you what you have to do. In your own way you will reach out and connect with him. It is then that you will understand the special gift you have to help another person to heal. You will also discover that in helping someone else you have helped yourself toward greater healing and continued growth. As is true of love, the more you give, the more you receive."

I like the term "wounded healer." There is a special healing touch which belongs only to those who have been wounded.

Prevention

(It's still worth a pound of cure any day!)

Set priorities. Make a list of all the tasks you perform. After making the list, read through and think about each item. Star those that are essential (going to work, grocery shopping, paying bills, child care, housework, etc.). Check those that are important to you (weekly bowling, singing in a group, attending your child's school events, seeing friends, etc.). Consider the remaining items to be unimportant. Cut them out of your life. Be very careful before you say "yes" to any more responsibilities. Say "no" to things that will overload your stress budget. If you have a tendency to completely fill your calendar, block some time out for relaxation. Remind yourself that relaxation is not an extravagance, but rather an essential part of life.

Manage your time well. An excellent, highly readable guide to both priority setting and time management is the book *How to Get Control of Your Time and Your Life*, by Alan Lakein. When time is not well managed, stress is too often the result. However, when people manage time well, they frequently experience the fulfilling sense of being in control of their lives.

Practice good nutrition and cut back on caffeine to avoid any extra "jitters."

Balance hassles with uplifts

In the July, 1981 issue of Psychology Today, Richard S. Lazarus shared his research that resulted in a list of the top ten hassles and top ten uplifts of middle-class men and women. He recommended offsetting hassles by incorporating the uplifts into one's life. As you read this list, think of your own hassles and uplifts.

Hassles	Uplifts
1. Concern about weight	1. Relating well with spouse or lover
2. Health of a family member	2. Relating well with friends
3. Rising prices of common goods.	3. Completing a task
4. Home maintenance	4. Feeling healthy
5. Too many things to do	5. Getting enough sleep
6. Misplacing or losing things	6. Eating out
7. Yard work or outside maintenance	7. Meeting responsiblities
8. Property, investment, or taxes	8. Visiting, phoning, or writing someone
9. Crime	9. Spending time with family
10.Physical appearance	10. Home pleasing to you

A similar idea is expressed by researchers at the Geisinger Clinic in Danville, Pennsylvania. They recommend that people think of themselves as a battery. You can spend your energy on life's tasks as much as you want (taking your special needs into account) as long as you energize yourself an equal amount. Balance your outputs with your inputs. Balance your energy drains with energizers!

Evaluate

Periodically list your stressors and your energizers. You are the only one who can keep them in balance. And you can only keep them in balance if you are aware of them.

Evaluate the effectiveness of your coping methods. Do you feel better? If you feel better, that is, less stressed, then perhaps you have dealt successfully with your stress. However, feeling better cannot be the only measure of successful stress management. Some people say they feel better after getting drunk or abusing their spouse. It is important that your stress management techniques yield positive and healthy benefits for you and those close to you. The goal is to have an overall positive impact on your well-being.

Knowledge

Continue on your own to seek more information on stress and its successful management. I have especially enjoyed the insights of Dr. George Vaillant, who has studied how people adapt to the changes in life. He recommends the following coping methods: altruism (giving of yourself to help others), sublimation (directing your energy into hobbies and other worthwhile pursuits), and humor.

I suggest the following books for more information on stress and well-being:

Stress/Unstress by Keith Sehnert.

Books by Jane Brody.

Feeling Good by David Burns, M.D.

The Power of Positive Thinking by Norman Vincent Peale.

The Gift of Hope by Robert Veninga.

In your knowledge gathering, seek to understand yourself better. Dr. Alan Marlatt of Washington University encourages self-awareness in his work on the psychology of relapse (re-starting a negative behavior). His recommendations include:

1. Know your high-risk situations, those which most commonly cause you to feel stressed.

2. Plan for high-risk situations by deciding ahead of time what stress management methods you will use. *See yourself in the high-risk setting, successfully using your chosen positive behavior to manage the stress it causes.*

3. See your progress on a continuum. If you slip occasionally, realize that it was only a temporary lapse and not a total relapse. People fail when they view their challenge as an all or nothing, win or lose process. Everyone "slips" from time to time. Forgive yourself. Then, keep moving forward.

A tool box for stress

View all of these techniques as if they were tools. You now have a whole tool box full of tools for stress management. Some will be useful in specific situations but not all the time. You choose which tool or tools will suit your unique needs at different times. A hammer can't do what a saw can do. Remember that as you choose your stress management tools. If one doesn't work, try another. But, also remember that they are *only* tools. Just as a hammer and saw cannot make furniture by themselves, neither can these stress management tools benefit you unless you *use them*. Perhaps the most important advice comes from the Ohio Mental Health Association: GUTS, or "Get Underway. Try Something!

And here's a great bit of advice for avoiding undue stress:

> We must try to take
> life moment by
> moment. The actual
> present is usually pretty
> tolerable, I think, if
> only we refrain
> from adding to its
> burden that of the
> past and the
> future. How
> right our Lord
> is about
> sufficient to the day.

C.S. Lewis

Letter to an American Lady

Summary

* Stress is an inevitable part of everyone's life. If you can cope successfully with the stresses of life, then you are in control.

* Having a disease adds stress to life, and it also makes it more important that you learn and use successful coping techniques.

* Stress is not an event. It is our perception of the event.

* If you are not making progress in managing the stress of your disease, seek professional counseling.

* Stress is like a violin: If violin strings have no stress (tension) then the violin can provide no music. But if too much stress is applied to the strings they snap.

* Know your stress signals — the feelings or behaviors that let you know stress is taking its toll on your well-being.

* Know where the stress comes from in your life, control the controllable sources of stress, and seek out healthy ways of coping with the remaining stress.

* Try various techniques for coping with stress, remembering that successful stress management requires preventive techniques as well as techniques to lessen the damage from temporary, major sources of stress. Build a tool box full of stress management techniques, and become a master craftsperson with your tools.

Reflection Questions

1. List the major sources of stress in your life today.

2. Decide which are controllable. Write a brief statement describing what steps you will take to control each controllable source of stress.

3. List each of the remaining "uncontrollable" stresses in your life. Next to each, list the technique you will use to cope with it.

4. List the Hassles and Uplifts in your life. (Use separate piece of paper.)

Hassles   Uplifts

After looking at your hassles and uplifts, decide if your life is in or out of balance. Describe below the action(s) you can take to get your life back in balance.

Chapter 6

Insights Into Solution Finding

Y our second-grader is home from school with the flu, but you have to teach class today.

Your car breaks down and you have to get to work.

You're short $500 for next semester's tuition.

The phone rings, the macaroni boils over, and the dog throws up, all at the same time.

You've been invited on a three-day canoe trip, but you need to follow a special meal plan and do several insulin injections and blood tests every day to control your diabetes.

You've got 20 people invited to your home for Christmas Eve, and that's the day you're scheduled for renal dialysis.

Problems confront everyone, every day. Some seem rather simple: "How will I get my car repaired?" Others seem quite complex: "How can I continue to enjoy life now that I have cancer?" But whether the problems are simple or complex, the approach to finding a solution is essentially the same. This chapter will explain the philosophy of solution finding and will present a practical, step-by-step approach you can use to solve problems in your life.

Desire, Determination, and Perseverance

The most basic philosophy of solution finding is that it is necessary to really concentrate on finding solutions. That is why I chose to use "solution finding" in the title of this chapter rather than the traditional "problem solving." One of the reasons some people fail at problem solving is that they become so caught up with the problem that they never find their way to the solution.

The people who are most likely to find solutions are the ones who have a strong *desire* to do so. The person who does not have much desire to go to work may view a sick child or broken car as a good excuse to stay home. The person who has a tremendous desire to go to school will find a way to earn or borrow the money for tuition. If there is a solution to a particular problem, it will be found by the person who desires to find it, the person with an "I can" attitude.

Here is a story that shows the contrast between a problem keeper and a solution finder:

I taught summer school once when I was an English teacher. The basic problem for all of the students in the summer school program was that they were non-participators. So, one of our culminating activities was a three-day canoe trip. For the canoe trip to work, everyone would have to do his or her share of cooking, wood gathering, paddling . . . "participating."

After weeks of planning, we met very early one morning to board the bus that would take us to the river. It was then that one of the students handed me a note from his father: "Please excuse Jim from the canoe trip. He cannot go because he has diabetes." Obviously, I was shocked that he felt he couldn't go on the canoe trip. "Jim," I said. "I have diabetes and I'm going!" Jim looked astonished. "Well," he sputtered, "what are you going to do with your insulin and syringes? If the canoe tips over they'll sink to the bottom of the river!" "They're in a plastic, air-tight container, Jim. If the canoe tips, they'll float."

> I really *wanted* to go on that canoe trip. My desire led me
> to figure out exactly how to do that. Jim really wanted
> to get out of going. He used his diabetes as an excuse to
> get out of any school-related activity.

Do some careful self-examination of your desires. Where do you get greater payoffs, from keeping your problems or from finding a solution? To nurture your desire to find a solution, keep reminding yourself of all the positive values you hold. It was love of family that fueled my friend Molly's desire to find a solution to her problem. Her renal dialysis fell on Christmas Eve day. Instead of giving up on the idea of entertaining her family that same day, she negotiated with the hospital and changed her dialysis to December 23.

Along with desire, other important elements of the philosophy of solution finding are *determination* and *perseverance*. Determination is the strength and energy you put into your effort. Perseverance is the duration of your effort, your "stick-to-itiveness." Determination becomes very real to me when I watch my nephew Eric take five minutes to tie his shoe. Cerebral palsy makes the otherwise simple task a great challenge for him. He has the class of determination about which Sir Winston Churchill spoke when he said, "Never give in. Never, never." And, perseverance adds her message: "Try again, and if that doesn't work, try again and again and again . . ."

> "Perseverance is not a long race;
> it is many short races one after another."
>
> Walter Elliot

No one has the strength to always find solutions without help. In the next two chapters we will examine support, the external and internal strengths that make desire, determination, and perseverance possible. With these important allies you can turn your attention to the practical approach to finding solutions.

Define your problem

"A problem well-stated is a problem half-solved."

Charles F. Kettering

In defining your problem, state it "well" by being both accurate and specific. If you state that your problem is your disease, you have not been specific enough. What is it about your disease that is a problem to you? Fear for the future? Frustration over the limitations it has imposed on your present life? (List these limitations specifically; mobility is not specific enough. A more helpful description of this limitation would be: I can't walk as fast as I want to, stairs are impossibly painful for me, or I'm embarrassed when people stare at me in public because I walk "funny.") Take time to specifically describe your problem. And, be accurate.

A simple example of an inaccurate definition of a problem is seen when someone defines their problem as diabetes after experiencing an embarrassing insulin reaction in the middle of a social event. By really looking at the situation objectively and honestly, that person would see that the real problem was a lack of preparedness. The reaction could have been avoided if meals were eaten on time, snacks were eaten as scheduled, exercise was figured into the day's eating and insulin schedule, and the person had carried something with which to treat the early signs of a reaction. This list of ways in which the reaction could have been avoided is an example of the second step in solution finding.

List all the things you can do about it

List all the things you can think of that might help solve your problem. If the problem is health-related you may need assistance from your medical team. But you may have enough knowledge to solve it yourself. People with lupus, multiple sclerosis, and many other diseases can experience a flare-up of their symptoms if their life becomes too busy or stressful. Sometimes they can solve this flare-up by making changes in their daily living. If this solution does not work, then the medical team is consulted.

The same is true for emotional or psychological problems. Sometimes you can solve them by giving yourself a pep talk or changing negative thoughts into positive ones. Other times you may need to turn to a professional counselor for help. Be sure to list *all* of your options. If one does not help, you need back-ups to try until you find the right one.

In brainstorming it is important not to limit yourself. List as many ideas as you can possibly think of. It is from that kind of a list that you will not only find "a" solution, but many solutions. Throughout life we are confronted with the same problems. To keep solving them we need plenty of reinforcements: solutions backing up solutions.

Since healthy eating is an important goal for everyone, let us use the challenge to doing so as an example in brainstorming solutions. The specific challenges to eating nutritiously are commonly overeating and making poor food choices. Following is the beginning of some brainstorming:

—in a restaurant, order smaller portions
—at home, serve plates instead of "family style"
—eat only what you should, then clear your plate
—eat only what you should, then heavily salt what is left on your plate
—concentrate on the atmosphere of the restaurant including decor, music and conversation.
—at home, get involved with family conversation and slow down your eating
—at a restaurant request that the meat portion be halved before it's brought to you with one half placed immediately into a doggie bag.
—choose dining companions with a similar interest in healthful, sensible eating (when you can)
—select restaurants carefully avoiding the 'all you can eat for one price' variety

—at home, make only as much as you and your family need, so that there are no 'seconds'

—if a recipe does make more than your family needs, put the leftovers into the refrigerator or freezer before you even sit down to eat.

—immediately after eating, brush your teeth so as to remove the taste of food from your mouth

—plan an activity to begin shortly after the meal so that your thoughts will naturally move to that activity and not dwell on food

—do not buy junk food or allow it in your home

—when bored, clean a closet, call a friend, go for a walk. Do anything except eat.

—when stressed look at your list of positive coping techniques. Use them, not food.

If you find it difficult to brainstorm alone, then do it with a friend, a support group, a member of your medical team or anyone with a similar interest.

Take action and evaluate

Now that you have a list of numerous options, start trying them. Evaluate as you do this. Is the problem getting solved? If so, you have successfully carried out the process. If not, try another of your options. If you are not finding effective solutions, go to your support system for assistance before you become discouraged. Here is an illustration of how this process works:

> **Problem:** "All I think about is my heart. I'm afraid to do things. I'm afraid that at any moment I will have another heart attack. I am consumed by myself and feel my life is out of balance."

Options:

1. I will replace my fearful thoughts with positive thoughts.

2. I will get busy with my hobbies so I won't be so wrapped up with my health.

3. I will express my concerns to my doctor.

Solution #1: No matter how many positive thoughts I give myself, that nagging fear is always there and returns day after day. I'll go to another option.

Solution #2: Even though I truly enjoy my hobby of woodworking, I could do it with my eyes closed. It just doesn't provide me with enough distraction to overcome my anxiety.

Solution #3: I visited my doctor and openly discussed my concerns. She gave me some helpful information about cardiac rehabilitation, which relieved some of my fears. Then, she recommended that I visit a counselor. I did, and it helped me regain a healthy perspective. My sense of well-being has definitely improved. Now I am finding that solutions 1 and 2 are helping me to hold on to my sense of balance in life.

Solving this problem was fairly simple, but it required a purposeful approach on the part of the individual. The person defined the problem, described three possible solutions, and then tried each to find which worked. Let's look at how the same process can work in a more complex example:

> **Problem:** "I'm worried. I've lost my job and I'm afraid that I won't find another. My worrying is causing me so much stress that my diabetes is often out of control. On top of that I'm coping with my stress by eating more than I should, adding to my diabetes control problems. I just can't see my way out of this!"

This person is so overwhelmed by the complexity of his problems that there is a real danger that he may not even be able to list possible solutions, much less act on them. When a problem gets as complex as this one, you must break it down into components. In *How to Get Control of Your Time and Your Life*, Alan Lakein recommends the "Swiss cheese" approach to problem solving. He advises that you break a problem down into smaller parts and then begin to work on one small part at a time. In this way you gradually make enough "holes" in the larger problem to make it fall apart, and it is resolved. Our friend has decided to take this approach to finding the solution to his problem.

Problem: "My basic problem is worry."

1. Worrying about finding a job.
2. Worrying that family and friends will think of me as a loser if I don't get another job real soon.
3. Worrying about the effect this stress is having on my diabetes.
4. I'm really frustrated that I'm coping so poorly. I know better. I just can't seem to get my life together!"

Options for worrying about finding a job: I will talk sense to myself. Lots of people lose jobs and then not only find new ones but even find jobs they like better than the one they lost. I really don't need to worry about finances yet. My wife has an excellent job and her income can sustain us until I find a job. I'll apply for a teaching job at all the schools close to us. I'll also look outside the teaching profession. My skills can be put to use elsewhere. To bolster my self-confidence for the job hunt, I'll attend community college seminars on resume writing and interviewing.

Options for worrying about what friends and family will think: I will again talk sense to myself. My family and friends are well aware of the general trend of declining enrollments in schools. It was my lack of seniority and not a lack of competence that caused met to be laid off. They know that. I will ask for their support. If they were in my shoes they'd want my support.

Options for worrying about the effects of stress on my diabetes: I will talk with my doctor and get advice on how to deal with these flare-ups as well as how to manage my stress more positively.

Options for my frustration at coping poorly: I'll get together with Steve and talk about how I feel. He always has a unique way of seeing the positive side of things, and he went through a job change just last year. Also, I'll attend the support group at the diabetes association. Those people always inspire me to believe in my ability to cope well.

I will set a goal of spending at least two hours each day calling around and checking out leads on jobs. And as a reward, I'll visit a a museum or go to an afternoon movie each week; this is the time for me to do all those things I daydreamed about during those long afternoons at work. I will forgive myself for past weaknesses at coping. I will give myself positive messages.

I can cope.

As our friend moved toward the solution phase of this process an interesting thing had already happened: he was worrying less. Just laying out his problem in small parts and planning options for solving each helped make it all manageable. He began to feel more in control of the situation. He then realized that his stress had immobilized him. Because he was feeling less overwhelmed, he was able to get moving on some of those solutions. Using the "Swiss cheese" approach he acted on one option after another and solved his problems one by one. Now, his worry has all but disappeared.

Sure there have been setbacks, especially the time he ran into some old pals from college who were having a business lunch to discuss a shared venture between their two companies. Hearing them talk so enthusiastically about their careers and then having to explain that he was out of work was *so* hard. He almost collapsed into self-pity. He cried a little and laughed a little, and then picked himself up and swore that one year from that day he would have lunch at the same restaurant, only this time as a happily employed, healthy person. All of the energy he had put into worrying, he is now putting into finding a new job and balancing his life. And not only is he feeling much better inside, he is a self-confident person on the outside—a fact he projects strongly in his job interviews.

Be logical instead of emotional

An important part of effective problem solving is the ability to be logical rather than emotional. Obviously, problems can cause an emotional response in anyone. Deal with the emotion until you can view youre problem from a logical rather than emotional perspective. One of the most amazing examples of someone who can *quickly* get into a logical perspective is a friend of mine who knew moments before he was rear-ended that the accident was about to occur. Steve saw the car approaching him very fast as he looked in his rearview mirror. Instead of getting into a panic, he immediately slid down in his seat and supported his neck on the back of his car seat. There was no way he could prevent the accident from happening, but his cool, logical problem solving prevented him from receiving serious whiplash.

Quality of Life

The broad, overall issue in solution finding is to achieve and maintain a quality of life that takes into account both the demands of your disease and the dreams you have for your life. Whenever a problem arises and threatens your quality of life, put it through the solution-finding process: Define your problem, break it down if it seems complex, list your options, take action, and evaluate. To ignite your spirit of determination, remember the thought of Eleanor Roosevelt:

> You gain strength, courage and confidence by every experience in which you really stop to look fear in the face ... You must do the thing which you think you cannot do.

Solving the challenges of a chronic disease

Some examples of finding solutions to problems common to people with a chronic disease may help you make a realistic assessment of your problem:

Case History - Bob Walters

Bob Walters visited his doctor for a routine, quarterly diabetes check-up. His blood test indicated that Bob's diabetes had been poorly controlled. Bob's doctor asked him, "How have things been going for you? Are you aware of any problem that would explain your diabetes being out of control?"

Definition of Problem: Bob defined his problem this way: "Diabetes places such heavy demands on our lifestyle that I'm afraid my wife just isn't able to do all the necessary meal preparation." The doctor asked Bob to bring his wife to the next appointment.

New Definition of Problem: As the doctor spoke with Bob and his wife she sensed a tremendous amount of friction in their relationship. Not only did they speak abruptly to each other, they argued openly about their eating habits. Mrs. Walters insisted that she provided the meals she had been taught to prepare for Bob. She accused Bob of uncontrolled snacking. To the doctor, it was quite apparent that diabetes was a problem secondary to their marital problems.

Moving Toward a Solution: The doctor recommended counseling for the Walters. They agreed, and as they progressed through counseling and rehabilitated their relationship, Bob's diabetes management improved.

Continued Solution Finding: Some months later when his diabetes was out of control, Bob was able to analyze the situation himself, and he realized that stress at work was his real problem. He realized he was coping with stress by eating, causing his diabetes to go out of control and causing him to gain weight, which was making him lose self-esteem. When Bob learned new, more positive coping methods he found the motivation and support to use them. Then he noticed three outcomes of his new behavior: he was controlling his diabetes well, he had achieved a healthy weight, and he felt better about himself as a person.

Case History - Marie Landini

Marie Landini has arthritis. It is very important that she do daily stretching exercises to retain mobility in her joints. Her doctor told her that the exercises would be painful at first, but that it was absolutely necessary to go through full range of motion daily. Marie not only failed to make progress in mobility, she actually lost mobility. When her doctor noted this, he asked Marie if she was faithfully doing her exercises.

Definition of Problem: Marie reported that it was sometimes so painful that she stopped. The doctor then asked her to demonstrate how she did the exercises. He observed that Marie arched her back and did many adaptive movements with her body, making the exercises almost worthless. They discovered two problems: the pain was causing her to quit too soon, and her technique of exercising was incorrect.

Moving Toward a Solution: The doctor referred Marie to a physical therapist who helped Marie practice her exercise technique. The therapist also gave her a videotape to take home to use as an instructional aid while she did her exercises, and he recommended that she place a full length mirror next to the television so she could compare her technique to that of the instructor. Seeing it done right helped Marie make sure her technique was correct. The videotape also helped distract Marie from the pain. She was able to hold her stretches longer than when she exercised alone. This helped her discover that when she was not able to watch the videotape she could do other things to distract herself, such as reading, watching television, or listening to music while she exercised.

Case History - Dan Hankinson

Dan Hankinson had a heart attack at the age of 47. When he left the hospital, he received instructions on how he should eat, exercise, and manage stress. In a follow-up visit to his doctor, Dan was still very much overweight, his cholesterol level was not declining, and he seemed depressed.

Definition of Problem: When Dan's physician asked him how he was doing, Dan said, "I don't know what my problem is. I understand very well what to do and why I need to do it, but I just can't seem to get myself going."

Moving Toward a Solution: Dan's doctor made two recommendations: join a support group of heart patients, and take a wellness seminar offered by the clinic, since virtually all the lifestyle recommendations of the wellness program would help Dan. His doctor felt that the wellness program could reinforce not only the valuable information of a healthy lifestyle, but also the important philosophy that Dan's new lifestyle is one of good health and good sense.

Dan chose not to join the support group because he felt that one more evening away from his family would cause more stress than it could relieve. So, Dan's doctor recommended that he visit with another of his patients who was close to Dan in age, had also had a heart attack, but was doing very well making the lifestyle changes and feeling the benefits of increased well-being.

Better Definition of Problem: Dan's visit with the other patient helped him learn some practical information on overcoming his obstacles, and made him better able to define his own problem. He realized that when he went out for lunch with his co-workers he was eating poorly. He blamed this on the type of restaurants they usually went to and the fact that everyone else ordered high fat selections and he found it difficult to do differently.

Moving Toward a Solution: Dan gained reinforcement for a healthy lifestyle from the wellness program. And his new-found friend shared some practical suggestions with Dan, such as "Be the first to order, maybe they'll follow the leader and order healthier meals. Suggest another restaurant with healthier selections; tell your co-workers about your need for nutritious meals, be more assertive." To Dan's pleasant surprise there were several people he worked with who were interested in good health and who joined him in ordering a turkey sandwich on whole wheat bread for lunch. An even more pleasant surprise was to feel his depression lift away and be replaced by a new enthusiasm for life. And, on his next check-up his doctor congratulated him on the health improvements he was making.

Case History - Karen Moore

Karen Moore is a teacher. She was diagnosed with liver cancer and spent months being very ill and undergoing vigorous therapy. She had to take a leave of absence from teaching. She became very depressed but sensed that her depression was not associated with a fear of dying. Karen's strong religious faith helped her regard death as a new beginning, rather than the end of life. This strong conviction left her confused about her depression. She sought the source of her problem by visiting with her pastor.

Definition of Problem: In visiting with her pastor Karen came to realize that her depression was linked to her frustration at not being able to fulfill her mission in life. Karen had been an outstanding teacher for more than 30 years. Teaching was her life. She defined her worth as a person within the context of teaching; she felt God had called her to teach.

Karen's pastor helped her realize that she had defined her mission too narrowly. His questioning and thoughtful listening helped Karen redefine her mission more broadly, as giving love. One of the ways she did that as a teacher was by appreciating the value in each of her students and nurturing individuals by pointing out their values to them. Her pastor suggested that until she could return to teaching she should find another way to fulfill her mission.

Moving Toward a Solution: Karen made a list of as many friends as she could think of. Then, she wrote next to each name something she appreciated about that person. She occupied her time each day by calling or writing friends to express this appreciation and love. Her days were also spent receiving calls and letters from the friends whom she had reached out to, expressing their appreciation for her friendship. Her depression lifted and she experienced the peace and contentment that comes when a person knows she is fulfilling her mission in life.

Apply the practical suggestions and inspirational messages of these case histories to help you find solutions to your problems. Keep in mind that the foundation of this process is *Belief, Desire and Action.* All of the belief and desire will do you no good unless you take action!

"To reach the port of heaven we must sail,
sometimes with the wind and sometimes against it,
but we must sail, not drift or lie at anchor."

Oliver Wendell Holmes

Summary

* To solve problems, concentrate on finding solutions, not on reasons to keep the problem.

* The person with a desire to find solutions will; the person without that desire will find excuses not to solve a problem.

* Determination is the strength and energy you put into finding solutions, trying them, and evaluating them.

* Perseverance is the duration of your effort, the ability to stick to it until the problem is solved.

* Start out by defining your problem, being accurate, specific, and honest with yourself. If the problem seems complicated, break it down into as many little problems as you can.

* List all the things you can do about your problem or the little parts that make up your complex problem.

* Take action on each of the solutions that seem appropriate. Give it an honest chance and then evaluate the situation to see if your problem is solved. If not, try another solution, and another until you find the one that works.

* Your goal in solution finding is to achieve and maintain a quality of life that reflects both the demands of your disease and the dreams you have for your life.

Reflection Questions

1. What is the major problem reducing your sense of well-being? State your problem accurately, specifically and honestly, breaking it down if it is complex:

2. Briefly describe why you want to solve your problem:

3. List all the ideas you can think of to solve your problem. (Make a long list, including even the "wild" ideas.)

4. Select the ideas that appeal most to you and list them.

5. Take action on one of the options listed in #4.

6. Evaluate your action. If the problem is solved, tackle the next part of it or go on to another problem. If the problem is not solved, try another option from #4.

Getting the Support You Need

F inders keepers, losers weepers! Do you remember that childhood chant? It leads into a discussion of support, another important element of a healthy life. Once you have found and developed the skills necessary to help you live well, you will want to *keep* them. Finders become keepers through on-going support. It is support that helps you to keep:

Viewing life as the pursuit and maintenance
of well-being,
Taking control of your self-image and how you
relate to others,
Getting motivated and staying motivated,
Adapting to life's continual changes,
Coping well with life's stresses,
Finding solutions,
Activating your physician within, and
Enjoying life while you "keep on keeping on."

Getting the support you need is a never-ending process, but once you understand and become good at techniques for helping others to help you, it becomes a natural and enriching part of a healthy life.

Support is as basic a need to human beings as a strong foundation is to a tall building. Knowing that the people you love, love you, is part of that support. Feeling accepted by your friends and co-workers is supportive. Receiving help at a time of need is the kind of support that has woven the very fabric of this country. It is support that gives people strength to face and to cope with the many challenges of life. As with all of the other life skills discussed in this book, support must be studied, observed, applied, and evaluated.

The study of support takes me back to my first job out of school. I was an English teacher and one of the classes I taught was American literature. Each semester I would ask my classes, "What quality is it that makes us American? What is the 'American character?'" The students invariably answered by saying that we are survivors. In explanation they would describe the early pioneers and their efforts to settle in the West. As the pioneers settled they did so in communities, not alone. They had neighbors. They built a town. They knew that if their barn ever burned, neighbors within a 50-mile radius would be there to help rebuild the barn. They felt supported.

The pioneers knew a wonderful quality of support:

You do not need to make use of support to be strengthened by it.

Their strength came from just knowing they had support. They did, however, make good use of it. They got together frequently with neighbors to work, worship, and socialize. Each positive gathering affirmed their feeling of support and strengthened them individually and collectively.

Challenges hit them. Fire destroyed homes, barns, livestock, and crops. Weather and insects ruined crops some years. Disease hit and people died: old people, fathers, mothers, children. Desperate, tragic challenges. And, challenges of frustration: Harsh winters kept people from seeing one another. A teacher moved away and suddenly there was no one to teach the children. The miracle of it all is that people survived. Most importantly, and the message we can learn most from, is that they didn't just survive physically. They survived emotionally, psychologically, and spiritually. In fact, many became stronger, wiser, gentler, and more thankful than ever for all they had.

The pioneers had trials, tragedies, and challenges. So do we. They survived and even thrived. So can we. Support helped them, and support can help us. In fact, the pioneers made use of all the life skills discussed in this book. They adapted, coped, solved problems, believed in a better tomorrow, used music and dancing to relieve stress, found the motivation to *get* going, and nurtured the support they needed to *keep* going.

We can be inspired by these pioneers as well as from modern day pioneers. Throughout history there have been frontiers to explore and conquer. A chronic health challenge is such a frontier. Researchers are continually seeking better treatments and cures to conquer disease and disability. That is their role as pioneers. We who have the diseases and disabilities are pioneers in the sense that we seek to live well with these challenges. We can conquer, if not the physical aspect, the psychological and spiritual challenges of our life.

I had the great privilege of working with a group of modern day pioneers who taught me a great deal about living well with a health challenge. They were parents of children who have diabetes. Although they did not have the disease themselves, they had to cope with it and teach their youngsters positive coping techniques.

My observation of these wonderful people gave me two important insights into how some people live well with their challenges: through practicality and faith. Many of these parents were from rural areas. They still face some of the challenges faced by the early pioneers: crop failure, loss of livestock due to disease, the windswept loneliness of Minnesota winters. But they too survive. I believe these people survive because they take a practical approach to life, and, each has a strong sense of faith.

This group of parents was meeting to support each other in techniques of positive parenting. Through positive parenting —encouragement and teaching by example rather than criticism and force—we believe parents provide the nurturing and support that children need to become strong, self-responsible, happy adults who cope positively with their challenges.

One of the specific topics one mother brought up was the ability to "let go" of one's child. It is difficult for any parent to know when and how to give children increased responsibility. This woman shared a remarkable experience with us. She told us that recently one of her sons had married. On the wedding day another of her sons was killed in an automobile accident. With tears just very gently rolling down her cheeks and with a peaceful expression on her face, she smiled and said, "I had to let go of two of my boys that day."

Later when we discussed the various families' acceptance of diabetes, it was this same beautiful woman who said, "Life has bumps and bruises but you go on. You make it." Underlying her message was a clear expression of faith that there would be a better tomorrow. It was quite clear that her strength, which was also exhibited by others in the group, came from the support of her family, friends, medical team, community, and God.

Those are generally recognized as basic sources of support: family, friends, the good "Doc," neighbors, and a power greater than ourselves. This chapter will cover four of those basic sources of support: family, friends, community (this includes neighbors, co-workers, and members of groups to which you belong), and medical. Spiritual support is covered in the next chapter.

As these various sources of support are discussed, reflect upon the support you currently have. Identify areas of support you would like to strengthen. The chapter will close with specific techniques you can use to get that support.

Family support

Families are frequently a strong sense of support. When one family member is in need, the whole family rallies to the aid of their brother/sister/parent/spouse/child. The strongest demonstration of support usually occurs at the initial diagnosis of the disease. Family members are attentive, encouraging, helpful. Quite commonly, however, this support falls off with time. People once again become consumed by the challenges of their own lives and may withdraw from the active support they were giving to their family member in need.

By their very nature, chronic health challenges do not go away. What happens when the support is gone ... but the challenge stays? Naturally, different people have different experiences. Some report that their family support has never waivered, others feel a sense of loss of family support. When we perceive a lack of support, we must look for ways to get support. But before you can ask for support you must understand what you mean by support. For some it is a nonchalant attitude from family members, for others it is an intense involvement. For me it has been a combination of active support and simply ignoring my diabetes. I very much appreciated being treated like a "normal" person by my family, but I also appreciated their occasional recognition of my situation.

My brother picked on me mercilessly, never treating me as if I needed to be treated any differently than any "kid sister." Then, out of the blue he would let me know he understood what I lived with.

When I was in ninth grade my brother was a senior in high school. One day he had to give a speech in English class on a subject of his choice. He chose to give his talk on diabetes. Like many ninth-graders I was in awe of twelfth-graders. I was very interested in what Pete would be telling his class about diabetes, because it seemed as though he would be saying it about me. I learned later that, among other things, Pete told the class that "People with diabetes are actually better citizens because they have to be very well-disciplined." Wow! My big brother said that about *me!* What tremendous support it was having that wonderful brother during those growing years.

My mother has certainly been the strongest, most consistent member in my support system. When I was first diagnosed it was she who made it seem that my diabetes was to be a blessing to our whole family. When I wanted to go to scout and church camps, Mother went along to work in the kitchen and pull weeds in the yard. She managed to achieve a perfect balance between providing me the support I needed without becoming overly protective and making me feel I'd never be able to make it without her. The only time I saw her was when I dashed over to her room to do my shot or when I passed through the cafeteria line and was "mysteriously" handed a plate with all the proper food exchanges. I knew that someday I would be managing all that for myself, but I really appreciated her helping me with it then.

Mother's support took other forms once I left home. When I went away to college she sent me the following poem:

> The rift in the chest of a mountain,
> The twist in the trunk of a tree
> The water-cut cave in the hollow
> The rough, rocky rim of the sea . . .
> Each one has a scar of distortion
> Yet each this sermon to sing
> "The presence of what would deface me,
> Has made me a beautiful thing."

What loving, nurturing support from a mother to a daughter! Years later it was to sustain me even more when my precious baby was injured and I helped him to accept his scars.

The support I receive from my husband and son is similar in that they are casual but concerned. We have worked out a system with which we are comfortable. It works for all of us. When my blood sugar is low and my disposition suffers, my son has learned to leave me alone until my blood sugar becomes normal. And, when he has his moments of crankiness, I've learned to give him a bit of breathing room and time to get back into balance.

Reflect on the ways in which your family is supportive of you. Think too of the ways in which you wish they were more supportive. For now, identify these two aspects of family support.

Social support

Most of the people outside of our family come under the category of "social supports." They include neighbors, co-workers, fellow members of organizations, and, the most important of the social supports, friends.

When our son was six years old he was faced with a major operation. The surgeon wanted to operate before John turned seven or eight. We sought advice from John's wonderful pediatrician on the timing of John's surgery with respect to his total well-being. We wanted to know not only when would be a good time in terms of physical considerations, but also in terms of John's psychological and emotional well-being. His response was, "Tell me about John's social supports. How does he feel about school? Does he have friends with whom he enjoys some good, imaginative play? Does he have good buddies? He'll be out of commission for awhile. Are his friends flakey or are they the sort who will be there ready to play as soon as John's ready? My chief concern is social support."

The scientific community has studied the impact of social

support and has reached the same conclusion our grandmothers did:

Friends are an important part of a healthy, happy life.

Not only do people enjoy friendships on a daily basis, they also derive great support from knowing they have the kind of friends who will *be there* if needed.

Besides the specific support your friends can offer to help you with your unique situation, how would you characterize your social support needs? It is important that you define those needs so that you can start working to fill them. Here is how some people I have met in support groups have described the support they want from friends. *Study* their descriptions. *Apply* them to yourself.

Listening: I always feel "listened to" when I'm with my friends. That makes me feel better.

Patience: They know my limitations and my needs. They never make me feel like a burden but help me fill my needs very matter-of-factly.

Respect: They are ready to give physical assistance only when I ask for it.

Inspiration: They've made it successfully through either the same challenge or one similar in magnitude.

Distraction: They're always ready for fun and laughter. I can count on these friends to help me get my mind off my troubles.

Acceptance: They don't judge me; they make me feel loved and cared about "no matter what."

Cheerfulness: They're generally upbeat. They're optimistic people, and just being with them or talking with them on the phone gives me a boost.

Guidance: They love me enough to speak honestly and lovingly to me. They don't let me get away with feeling sorry for myself and getting stuck in self-pity. They help point me in a positive direction.

Now, *evaluate*. Is there a description or several descriptions that tell you how you like to get support from friends? Use them as a means to identify what you are looking for from each of your friends. It is perhaps a more serious friend who will prove to be the excellent listener. Your cheerful, upbeat friend may not be as good a listener, but you value him or her for lifting your spirits.

Also evaluate the way in which you ask for support. Would you want to support someone who asks the way you do? A sure way to turn off your supporters is to be whiney, demanding, or constantly negative. People have a tendency to finally stop asking "How are you?" when the only response they ever get is negative. Listen to and observe yourself.

If you feel that the friends you now have cannot meet all your social support needs, get involved in clubs or organizations where you can meet new friends. Remember that social support is a two-way street, and that to get the depth of support you need, you must be able to give support. For example, if you are a good listener, try asking a new friend to tell you about his or her life; it could be the start of a deep, trusting friendship.

Be open to receiving support from people you have not yet met. I received tremendous support from just such a friend.

A woman I knew died suddenly after what seemed to be a victorious recovery from a kidney transplant. Stephanie was in her twenties. Those of us who had been through any part of the struggle with her were stunned by her death. We thought that after all the trial and difficulty she had finally made it. Her funeral was particularly sad and I wept throughout it. I reflected upon what seemed an intolerable injustice. Stephanie had suffered terribly before and throughout her kidney transplant. She wanted so desperately to live. She made it through the transplant and was recovering beautifully. Suddenly she was gone.

I felt numb as I left the church following the funeral. As I walked down the street to my car I was greeted by a friend. I turned and saw that she was with a Laotian woman whom our church sponsors. The Laotian woman was very new to our country and spoke no English. I felt a bit awkward because of my tears. I explained to my friend that I had been to a funeral. Then, I looked at the other woman. I gestured toward the church, then helplessly looked back at her, trying to explain. As I looked into her face I saw my anguish mirrored in her eyes. She knew. Not only did she know that I was grieving for a friend, but she herself *knew* the same anguish. She had lost young friends in Laos. She had, in fact, left her mother and eldest son in Laos. She knew sadness, injustice, and she also knew peace.

That brief, wordless encounter began my healing. Although Stephanie's death still seems an injustice, I derived a small bit of peace when I realized that people do survive injustice. I felt connected with another human being who understood my pain and who had struggled with it and had come to her own peace.

Identify *who* your social supports are and *how* they fill your support needs.

Medical support

The next very important part of your support network is your medical team. The word "team" may not be familiar to you in describing your medical support. It describes all the people with whom you work to face your health challenge. Depending on your disease or disability, your team may include doctors, nurses, dietitians, counselors, secretaries, physical therapists, social workers, and anybody who works together with you in some aspect of your well-being.

Chronic means "marked by long duration." People with

chronic health problems face their challenges everyday, for a long time. Since it is impractical to confer with one's doctor everyday, the person with the health challenge must be knowledgeable enough to make many of the day-to-day decisions. That knowledge can come from your medical team as you participate with them in making decisions about your health. This means *you* are an important part of the team. Ultimately, it is *you* who must take charge of the day-to-day decisions and maintenance of your health and well- being.

Dr. Donnell D. Etzwiler, Director of the International Diabetes Center, is truly one of the great pioneers of the team approach to chronic disease management and of making the person with the disease a central part of the team. The educational programs of the International Diabetes Center are important not only because they are comprehensive in including all medical disciplines. They are also important to the families and health professionals who attend them, because they focus on living *well* with diabetes.

Now, let's examine the role of the medical team in promoting your well-being. As various aspects of medical support are described, identify the support you want and feel you are lacking.

The most obvious support from a medical team is the traditional role they play as healers. To receive the best advice you need a physician who is knowledgeable in your specific health challenge. An endocrinologist is a specialist in diabetes, a cardiologist in heart disease, a rheumatologist in arthritis and lupus, an oncologist in cancer. Make certain that your team is led by a thoroughly knowledgeable specialist in your area. If you choose a generalist such as a family practitioner or an internist, find out how equipped they are to manage your case. Some indicators of this might include: How many other patients with your challenge are in his or her practice? Who is he or she affiliated with? What updates has he or she attended recently? Does he or she have ready access to consult with an expert in your health challenge? From a knowledgeable medical team you can receive the support of excellent, up-to-date treatment.

The second form of support you can receive from your medical team is a comprehensive education in how to live well with your health challenge. I consider the gold standard for health education to be that offered at the International Diabetes Center and its affiliated centers. It goes beyond specific information about the diabetes and its treatment, to how best you can fit it into your family situation and all facets of your life.

The medical team can also help you to *problem solve*. That is, of course, help you to find your own solutions, not just solve the problems for you. The way this works best is for you to inform the appropriate member of the team about a particular problem you may be having. That person and perhaps others on the team then brainstorm solutions with you, and then you choose the solution that appeals to you.

To the person with hypertension who says she's having trouble restricting salt, a dietitian might suggest specific low-sodium products, several cookbooks, and a low-salt cooking class.

To the cancer patient who feels his family is treating him as if cancer is contagious, a counselor might recommend some excellent books on cancer, a well-run local support group that offers both information and support for patients and families, or even that the family come along to the next medical appointment and express concerns directly to the doctor.

To the person having a hard time relaxing while recovering from a heart attack, a nurse may suggest important stress management techniques, a different form of exercise, or perhaps a different sleeping pattern.

The members of your medical team can also give support by being good *role models*. It is difficult to take advice to stop smoking from a physician who smokes. And, it is inspiring and helpful when the physician who advises exercise is a regular exerciser. And the dietitian who eats the same way she tells me to eat truly convinces me that, "The diet recommended for people with diabetes is an excellent, healthy way to eat. Everyone should eat this way."

The communication of genuine *caring* is another way the medical team gives support. In the medical world they refer to the art versus the science of medicine. Knowledge and skill represent the science, caring and person-to-person relating demonstrate the art. In all the years I have been a consumer of medical services I have come to view caring as:

1. *Listening.* Real, honest-to-goodness, eye-contact, facial response, question-asking, interested, unhurried listening.

2. *Touching.* A genuine, laying-on-of-the-hands, I-care-about-you, you're-worthy-of-my-involvement touch.

3. *Responding.* A returned phone call, an answer to a question, a smile, a handshake or a hug, a caring one-human-being-to-another responsiveness.

The expression of *positive expectations* supports hope. The health care provider who communicates positive expectations gives a message of "I see positive energies in you. I know you can handle this." The German poet and philosopher Goethe expressed this when he said:

"When we treat a man as he is, we make him worse than he is.

When we treat him as if he already were what he potentially could be, we make him what he should be."

Goethe

Numerous studies have shown that people rise or fall to meet the expectations of the influential people in their lives. The health care provider who is upbeat and positive about your future is the one who promotes well-being rather than illness.

Blessed is the person whose medical team takes a wellness

approach to the management of the health challenge. This is the best of three basic approaches: illness, prevention, and wellness. These different approaches can be placed on a wellness continuum that goes from minus 100 to plus 100.

-100...................... 0...................... +100
ILLNESS   PREVENTION   WELLNESS

The *illness* approach goes from -100 to 0, and is characterized by negative expressions like, "Since you have this disease you can expect the following deterioration of your health until you die." With this approach you wait until problems appear, then fix whatever can be fixed.

The *prevention* approach is right at 0, and encourages clients to have regular check-ups to catch problems as early as possible. Clients are taught what causes health problems and are encouraged to pursue behaviors designed to prevent problems.

The *wellness* approach expands from 0 to +100, and encourages people to take care of themselves so they can continue to live a happy, fulfilling life. This approach is characterized by the positive expectation of an enriching future. This approach has been extremely important to me. The illness approach is out of the question. But, I can't imagine taking the prevention approach either. I can't see myself getting out of bed in the morning, stretching, and saying, "Well, another day to prevent blindness and kidney failure!" As if that were a reason to live? It is the wellness approach to my diabetes that causes me to take four insulin shots a day, test my blood sugar four times a day, exercise, and follow a prescribed meal plan so that I feel well enough to enjoy my family, friends, and work.

My wonderful (carefully selected), wellness-oriented physician encourages my own wellness approach by asking questions about my life when we have appointments. He does not simply dwell on blood sugars and other physical aspects of my diabetes. This reinforces my own belief that the reason I work so hard to manage my diabetes is so I can enjoy life, not simply to prevent problems. This also reinforces my hope that I can prevent complications of the disease.

Your medical team members can help you study helpful information, apply it to your health situation, and evaluate the results on your well-being. They should be viewed as an ongoing source of support.

A support group is people who face a similar problem and are willing to share their successes and failures in dealing with it. The group provides social support and problem solving discussions. Support groups are usually led by a counselor or other medical professional, or they may be led by clergy or by a lay person who has received some training in leading a support group. If a group is made up of people who are living well with their challenge, it can provide the additional support of inspiration. If a group is made up of poor copers who enjoy complaining, it can reinforce problems instead of solving them. If you decide to seek support through a support group, ask your medical team to recommend one that is reputable and well-run.

The format for a successful support group is similar to the approach to solution finding: identify the problem, list your options, choose an option, and act. The philosophy for a group can be expressed in a simple creed: "We will accept one another, listen to one another, and care about one another. We will grow." Groups can be kept "on track" by reviewing the format and philosophy at the beginning of each meeting.

Now that we have done a preliminary evaluation of how people get support from family, friends and their medical team, evaluate *your* support. Which of the following statements describes in general how supported you feel right now?

I feel totally unsupported. I feel alone.
I feel supported in some areas of my life, but not in all.
I feel supported in most of the important areas of my life.

I feel totally supported.

Let's look at some techniques you can use to get that support.

Encouraging family and social support

In order to receive support it is frequently necessary to ask for it. You have defined the support you need or want, and now the next step is to actively seek it. Sometimes it is difficult to ask for support. Our culture encourages self-reliance and independence. People must work at being "interdependent." A healthy life is a *balance* of independence and dependence; that's interdependence. Sometimes I need you and sometimes you need me. That's healthy.

Mutual respect is the foundation from which family and social support arise. Interdependence comes out of mutual respect. It is an even larger issue of basic respect for life. It is an expression of the shared value of a fulfilling life, a recognition that a problem has placed that value in jeopardy, and a request for help from one human being to another.

Giving support is an action that follows mutual respect quite naturally. Look for opportunities to give support to the people from whom you would like to receive it. You can set the "tone" of a relationship through your spirit and acts of giving. Sending a pot of soup to a neighbor who has a house full of out-of-town guests is the sort of act that encourages a phone call or visit when *you* need it.

Gratitude and its most common expression, "Thank you!" are the cement that binds relationships. This positive reinforcement of positive behavior makes it more likely that the person will offer it again. Buy a stack of thank you post cards and postage stamps so that you're always ready. Reinforce every kindness with a thank you. Remember to express gratitude to your family, for they are most often neglected or taken for granted. Some people report that one of the positive aspects of their disease is the appreciation and expressions of love and gratitude it fostered among family members.

Communication is vital to the development of supportive relationships. We will examine three areas in communication: education, assertiveness, and listening.

Education of family members encourages cooperation (eating meals on time), alleviates or removes fear ("Nothing in life is to be feared. It is only to be understood." Marie Curie) and promotes understanding ("So that's why you feel like that following chemotherapy!"). Education of friends can provide you with the sort of support that removes obstacles. When our friends invite us to dinner they let me know what they'll be serving and what time it will be served. They understand that I need that information to plan for my insulin needs. How supportive that is!

Assertiveness as defined in *Your Perfect Right* by Alberti and Emmons is: "Behavior which enables a person to act in his/her own best interests, to stand up for him/herself without undue anxiety, to express his/her honest feelings comfortably or to exercise his/her rights without denying the rights of others."

Unassertiveness creates unnecessary pain and problems, for example, when a person with poor mobility neglects to tell friends and therefore is forced to walk many stairs for fear of being a burden, or when a person with digestive problems eats whatever the hostess serves, for fear of being impolite. Let your friends know what you need and why you need it. Keep interdependence in mind.

If you find yourself feeling uncomfortable about asking for what you need, pretend that the situation were reversed. Imagine that it is your best friend who has the disease or special requirements. Wouldn't you, as a friend, want to do everything you could to be supportive? Wouldn't you feel hurt if you found out that your friend had a special dietary need and had not told you when he or she ate at your home?

Whole books have been written on assertiveness. If you feel a special need to get help in this area, seek books and classes that teach assertiveness. Here are the basic guidelines to keep in mind:

1. Enter into assertive behavior only after giving yourself positive messages so that your attitude is positive. One such message is the definition of Alberti and Emmons. Memorize it and review it before expressing yourself.

2. Practice being assertive. It is a skill and won't come overnight. Practice in non-threatening situations with people with whom you feel comfortable. For example, when a friend calls and invites you to see a movie you don't care to see, practice your assertiveness skill by calmly and honestly expressing your feelings. "I'd like to go to the movie with you, but I don't really care to see that particular one. How about the one showing at the Lyceum?"

3. Be factual instead of emotional. You can talk about your feelings in a factual manner. Tone of voice (calm rather than whiney) helps you to keep the discussion factual. "I feel lonely when you never ask me how I'm getting along. When you know that I've been to the doctor I would feel so supported if you remembered that and inquired about it."

4. Rehearse it. Visualize yourself looking calm and in charge, then plan what you want to say. Find a quiet spot somewhere, where you can actually rehearse it.

Sometimes a supporter will be assertive on your behalf:

An acquaintance told me that his wife had had a mastectomy. He said she was doing very well, both physically and psychologically. Then, an amazing thing happened. His wife's tennis partners, in a misguided attempt to be supportive, found a new partner without asking her if she'd be able to play anymore. They assumed she could never play again and decided it would be easier on her if they simply replaced her. The woman's husband called the tennis partners and told them how vitally important it was to his wife's recovery that she have her tennis to look forward to. "She's almost ready to play again," he announced to the amazed women.

Listening is the other half of communication. What are your family's and friends' needs? Are they frightened by your disease or disability? Deal with that through education, taking them with you to one of your doctor visits, or to a counseling session. Listen to their general needs. Surely the disease or disability becomes a part of both your family and social life, and as such, it must be dealt with. But your family and friends still have their own needs that have nothing to do with your challenge.

It may be difficult to seriously consider a daughter's acne or a friend's broken car when you feel that your challenge is so much greater. Try to see their problems for what they are: problems in need of solutions. Share the steps in the solution finding chapter with them. In doing that you will have participated in mutual respect and promoted mutual support. You will experience a surge of emotional well-being if you do that. You will have risen above your illness to deal with the needs of another person.

Some friends will be more supportive that others. You can choose to gravitate to those who support you. But because we live with family members day in and day out, it is crucial to have their support. If you find that you and your family are simply unable to follow these guidelines to establish a healthy system of communication, then do seek help. Family counseling is a wise step in a very healthy direction.

It may take time for family counseling to help. I once heard someone say, "Oh, it isn't worth it. It'll probably take a year for us to iron out all our problems!" Ask yourself this: In one year would you prefer to have a healed and healthy family because you spent that year in counseling? Or would you prefer to still be in a broken or unhealthy family? Support comes in many forms, and counseling is one. Healthy people get the support they need. Choose to be healthy!

Encouraging medical support

Communication and cooperation are the basic ways in which we get the support desired from the medical team. The "Plan of Action" in the last chapter will serve as a good guide for your communication with your medical team. Basically, discuss the *goal(s)* of your treatment plan with your medical team and reach agreement on how those goals will affect your well-being. Then, honestly and openly discuss the obstacles you will have to overcome to achieve those goals. That's where problem solving comes in. With your medical team's expertise and experience and your knowledge of your own capabilities, you can find ways to overcome your obstacles. Finally, let them know what you feel you need for ongoing support (frequency of follow-up appointments, a phone call three days after beginning a new drug, etc.).

One of the best ways in which people can be cooperative members of their medical team is to become educated about their health challenge. We all are responsible for taking charge of our own well-being. We do that by seeking information, getting help understanding and applying the information to our own situation when necessary, and then making appropriate use of that information. To make the most of this process, you need to use assertiveness techniques to ask questions whenever you are unclear about something:

> Once when I had tendinitis I went to an internist. He advised me to take cortisone. Fortunately, I had heard that cortisone can cause diabetes to be more difficult to manage. So I asked the internist, "What about my diabetes?" He looked startled and asked "What diabetes?" Although my chart was right in front of him he had not noticed that I have insulin-dependent diabetes. He then prescribed a different drug, but I would have had problems if I had not spoken up.

Another aspect of a cooperative attitude is to realize that anyone can make a mistake. I believe that one of the reasons people are not more assertive with medical professionals is that they feel they are somehow super-human. They aren't. They make mistakes just like you and I do. We must not view them as gods, nor should we view them as enemies. We are all in this together.

We cannot expect the medical community to promote our health and well-being all by themselves. We must take responsibility. One of the ways we can do that is by asking questions when we do not understand, or by asking the reason for something they have recommended. They certainly ought to be able to answer our questions in language we can understand and justify their recommendations in terms of our treatment goals. In order to nurture a relationship of mutual respect and trust, learn how to ask your questions in an assertvie manner and not in an aggressive or passive manner. Here are some descriptions and examples of these varying communication styles:

Aggressive: When I think of only myself.
Passive: When I think of only the other person.
Assertive: When I think of both of us.
Let's apply each style to a specific situation:

Martha was in the hospital, and at regular intervals she was given two pills. Her doctor had explained what the drugs were, how often they were to be taken, and what effect they might be expected to have. One evening the nurse brought her the pill cup and inside she saw the two familiar pills and a third pill she did not recognize.

The *aggressive* approach to this situation might be: "What's the third pill? What's wrong with this hospital anyway? Are you trying to kill me?"

The *passive* approach would be to say nothing and simply take the pill, thinking, "I wonder what that third pill is? Oh well, they know best."

The *assertive* approach is to simply ask, "I recognize the iron pill and the benedryl, but what is the third pill?"

My most dramatic personal example of needing to assert myself occurred shortly before I was to be married. My physician told me that he thought it was fine if I got married, "But don't have children. Don't spread your genes around." Instead of simply taking his advice, I chose to go with my husband to a genetic counselor. He gave us facts that were extremely encouraging. Then, based on real information, my husband and I made the choice to have a child. The supportive medical team I chose to see me through my pregnancy did not include the ill-informed and thoughtless physician who advised me not to have children.

At the conclusion of *Anatomy of an Illness*, Norman Cousins recounts what he said to the doctor who had told him he would experience progressive paralysis. Cousins met him on the street ten years later. When the physician inquired about Cousins's recovery, Cousins replied, "It all began when I decided that some experts don't really know enough to make a pronouncement of doom on a human being. And, I said, I hoped they would be careful about what they said to others; they might be believed and that could be the beginning of the end."

This is not to suggest that we should not believe what medical professionals tell us. It does mean that we must filter all of what we are told and make our own educated as well as intuitive selection of what to believe.

Support yourself

Besides actively seeking support from others, be sure that you are supporting yourself. Seek support everywhere with the expectation that you will find it. Be creative in thinking of all the sources of support you have in your life. I feel supported by the college from which I graduated, Gustavus Adolphus College. The most important support comes from the values that guide the college and that reinforce my own values. Here is one sentence from the college's mission statement:

"Gustavus Adolphus College seeks to encourage a mature understanding of the Christian faith, service to others, sensitivity to community, an international perspective, and attitudes and behaviors that work toward a peaceful and free world."

How reinforcing it is to realize that the most meaningful values in my life transcend disease. Diabetes in no way prevents me from serving God, community and others.

The world is full of brave, strong, inspiring people. In January 1981, when the U.S. embassy in Iran was attacked and the people taken hostage, I heard a radio commentator say, "Sometimes hanging in there, surviving, is a form of heroism too." How true!

Helen Keller once said, "So much has been given to me that I have no time to ponder over that which has been denied." Think about that! How inspiring! Read the biographies of famous people. You will find that there were many difficult challenges in their lives.

Booker T. Washington said it so well: "I have learned that success is to be measured not so much by the position that one has reached in life, as by the obstacles which he has overcome while trying to succeed." Indeed. Without obstacles, where would the greatness of the human spirit be?

"We are not at our best perched at the summit; we are climbers, at our best, when the way is steep."

John W. Gardner

How amazing and inspiring are those people who suffer great pain and yet always find things about which they are thankful. Thanksgiving was made a national holiday in 1863. In the midst of the Civil War, one of the greatest tragedies of our country, Abraham Lincoln paused to dedicate a whole day to giving thanks.

Since it is thoughts that create our feelings, one of the best ways to support yourself is by giving yourself positive thoughts.

"Though we travel the world over to find the beautiful,
We must carry it with us or we find it not."

Ralph Waldo Emerson

When we give ourselves worthy thoughts, they become a part of us. I read about an 80-year-old woman who is blind. She made this insightful comment:

"People should furnish their minds well. If I have to sit alone, at least I can sit in my own well-furnished mind."

Ultimately, the support we need goes beyond the physical and the psychological to the spiritual. The next chapter turns to the spiritual force in your life, your Physician Within. We will look at nourishing that force.

If I had but three loaves of bread
I would sell one and buy hyacinths
For they would feed my soul.

The Koran

Before we can nourish that force, we must discover it.

Summary

* Support from others is as basic a need to human beings as a strong foundation is to a tall building.

* You do not need to make use of support to be strengthened by it.

* Your basic sources of support are family, friends and other social acquaintances, the members of your medical team, and your spiritual faith.

* Before you can ask for support from your family you must define yourself how you would like to be supported, whether casually or very intensely, or somewhere in between.

* Friends can provide different types of support, depending on whether each is a good listener, an inspiring example, or a cheerful spirit lifter. Likewise, you can provide support through your personality strengths. By giving support, you will be more likely to get support from friends.

* Successful management of most chronic health challenges requires a knowledgeable and coordinated medical team, each of whom can teach you about a specific part of your health needs and help you solve problems related to those needs. The medical team works best when you become knowledgeable enough to act as an integral member of the team.

* Management of a health challenge can be characterized by one of three basic approaches: Illness, in which you wait for problems to appear and try to fix what can be fixed; prevention, in which you have check-ups to try to catch things as early as possible and in which you follow specific behaviors because they may prevent problems, and; wellness, in which you take care of yourself so that you can live a happy, fulfilling life.

* A healthy life is a balance of independence and dependence on others. To encourage others to support you, nurture a

sense of mutual respect, give support to others, express gratitude at every opportunity, and communicate your support needs clearly and assertively.

* Assertiveness is thinking of yourself and the person with whom you are communicating; it is telling someone what you need and why you need it; it is asking questions or requesting an explanation, realizing that anyone can make a mistake.

* Seek support everywhere with the expectation that you will find it.

Reflection Questions

1. Make a list of your sources of support, and then evaluate
   each:

	Not supportive	Supportive	Very supportive
Family			
Social			
Medical			
Other			

2. Place a mark by those sources from whom you would like
   greater support. Then, write out specific action(s) you will
   take to encourage more support in your life.

3. List the ways in which you will *give* support to these sources of support.

List five people (famous or otherwise) you appreciate. Briefly describe one or two challenges in this person's life. Then, identify the quality in that person that you most appreciate and would most like to have.

	PEOPLE I APPRECIATE	CHALLENGES THEY FACE	QUALITY I LIKE
1.			
2.			
3.			
4.			
5.			

Discover Your Physician Within

> H ope is the thing with feathers
> that perches in the soul
> And sings the tune without the words
> And never stops at all.

Emily Dickinson

Hope is surely one word that could be used to describe the Physician Within. It is a source of support that will *always* be with you. The preceding chapter explained how to make the most of your external sources of support. This chapter deals with making the most of your internal sources of support. If and when the sources of support around you are not there when you need them or are not sufficient, you can draw on your internal support. You must have an internal source which, as the poem by Emily Dickinson suggests, "never stops."

This chapter will encourage you and help you to discover the most powerful force in your life, your spirit. It is the spiritual domain of your life that gives you *strength* to persevere in the face of life's most difficult challenges, *peace* in facing unanswerable questions, and a *joy* that mysteriously enters the heart.

Once you identify this force you need to figure out how to *activate* it and *nourish* it. Although this power source can be a person's most important support, many individuals ignore it or don't completely understand it. It is fairly easy for us to identify our external sources of support: family, spouse, friends, doctor, pastor, counselor, etc. But our internal source of support is not visible. You can *feel* its strength and support but you cannot see it. It is difficult for us to believe in something we cannot see. That is your greatest challenge, because it is *belief* that activates your Physician Within.

Your Physician Within is that force which you recognize as being greater than you are. No one can define it for you or describe what it will mean in your life. In this chapter I will share with you some of the discoveries others have made. I will share with you my personal understanding of my Physician Within. As you read these descriptions, hold a spiritual mirror up to yourself. Look into your soul. Discover. Then, prepare yourself to nourish and sustain the powerful, essential force that lies within.

We know that there is more to human beings than body and mind. There is also the spirit. Biology and psychology teach us about the body and mind, but there are a variety of resources for studying the spiritual aspect of life. The more organized and concrete resources include philosophy, literature, and religion. The most convincing resource, however, is experience. Sometimes we experience spirituality by observing others, and this can be convincing and helpful. However, it is your direct, personal experience that will be the most persuasive and valuable means of discovering your Physician Within.

Many experiences can contribute to your belief in this force, but it is often during life's darkest, most difficult moments that we discover or fully appreciate this wonderful, sustaining, never ending source of strength and comfort.

When our precious son was born I had had diabetes for 19 years. It was still the "Dark Ages" of diabetes management, in that blood glucose monitoring was not yet available to allow close control of blood glucose on a daily basis. So, my diabetes was not easily managed and the pregnancy was in the high-risk category, unlike today.

Thankfully, our son was born triumphantly healthy. However, he became the victim of a hospital mistake. He was slightly low in calcium at birth, and an IV solution of calcium was delivered at ten times the prescribed concentration. Our newborn was very seriously burned. He lost all the skin, fatty tissue, veins, and some of the nerves from his knee to his toes on one leg. A plastic surgeon performed split-thickness skin grafting, and John came home at age four weeks.

Several months later our life centered around our precious baby and the ongoing challenge of his injury. Although the skin graft was successful, it was contracting as John grew. His foot was being pulled up. He began seeing an orthopedic surgeon, who applied a new plaster cast to his leg each week. As the plaster dried the orthopedic surgeon applied great pressure downward so that the hardened cast would hold John's foot down. As one of the first casts was removed, we discovered that John's leg was swollen with a terrible infection. The graft had not healed adequately to be covered with a plaster cast. The pediatrician ordered X-rays, and we waited in anguish to learn whether the infection had invaded the bone. Thankfully it hadn't.

It was a difficult time for us, waiting for this nightmare to end. One problem after another surfaced. And although our attention was focused on John, other concerns arose. My husband Dale, a teacher, was aware that his school was facing severe budget cuts, and there was talk of layoffs. We didn't worry about these "might be's"; we had enough real problems demanding our attention.

It is during times of difficulty that we find comfort being able to talk with the people in our support system. But for the first time in my life I felt I couldn't go to my supporters. Although they loved and supported us in general, they could not support our decision not to sue the hospital. Our friends and family felt that we were wrong not to sue. One acquaintance even told me that I was a bad mother for not suing. She thought I ought to be concerned about providing for John's future through a cash settlement. We were concerned about John's future, but we would provide for his needs on our own.

Finally, we retreated from our support network and drew in toward our little family of three. We concentrated on doing what we had to do for John. The next decision was to put a fiberglass cast on his leg and leave a window over the graft area so that we could dress it and air could get to it. It was heavy and cumbersome. John couldn't lie down to sleep, so we placed him in his infant seat in his crib. He cried endlessly. I kept telling myself that he wasn't in pain, he was just crying because of the awkwardness and the frustration of not being able to really stretch out.

After two weeks, this cast was removed. When it was cut off I was horrified to discover a sadly misshapen little foot. The window cut-out had caused uneven pressure on John's foot and bent it grossly out of shape. My first thought was "All that crying WAS from pain. My baby has suffered so much!" I felt an intolerable pain. The surgeon shook his head and said, "We'll just leave casts off for awhile, now." I took John home.

When Dale got home that night I couldn't wait to unburden myself. The minute he walked through the door I began to tell of our dreadful experience and John's poor little foot. When I finally finished I realized that my husband looked dazed. His first words were, "I lost my job today."

It was at that very instant that I knew we were going to be fine. I felt a strange peace settle over me, which in light of the circumstances surely transcends normal understanding. Most importantly, I knew that a power greater than Dale and

I was in control and would take care of us and our son.

My Physician Within is God. He is always "there." He is within me at all times, but in order for me to derive strength and help I must place my trust in Him. This is another way of saying that it is *belief* that activates the Physician Within.

Look back on your life. When have you experienced that sort of inner peace and strength? Perhaps you are already very aware of how you define your Physician Within. Once you have truly experienced the power of your internal support, you will believe in it. Your own personal experience will help you to be specific in defining your Physician Within. Defining what you believe that force to be and what it means in your life are necessary steps that will enable you to gain the most support in times of greatest need. Sharing that feeling and observing other people's experiences with their inner force will reinforce your general belief in this spiritual power.

Many of us have found inspiration from the stories of American pioneers. We think of the spirit of America as a spirit of determination. Our ancestors seem somehow invincible. We tend to romanticize their hardships, though. We sometimes view their challenges as part of their exciting frontier life. But to receive true inspiration from the experiences we observe and learn about, we must view them realistically.

How do you suppose the pioneers really responded to the challenges and tragedies with which they were faced? Let's imagine a couple named Edward and Martha Anderson, a typical pioneer couple who travelled west and settled on some property they intended to farm. After spending all their money to buy the property, they discover that the land is rocky, the soil sandy, and there isn't enough water for their livestock. After tremendous efforts, working 18 hours a day seven days a week, they finally get the land cleared enough to raise just enough food to sustain them, but not enough to make any money.

After seven years Martha has had seven pregnancies, but only three babies survive. One evening after the children are asleep, Edward and Martha sit by the fire trying to keep warm. Martha's hands, numb with the cold, work awkwardly to patch for the fifth time a pair of child's trousers. "I'm tired, Edward," she says. "I don't know how much more I can take. When we decided to leave Virginia it seemed exciting and promising, but it has been only difficult. Why has this happened to us? The Jamiesons found property that is rich and fertile. They have prospered. It isn't fair Edward. Mrs. Jamieson has six healthy children. Four of our babies lie in the cold ground. Life is so unfair!"

That same conversation could have taken place in many pioneer homes. The hardships were dreadful. Everyone experienced feelings of discouragement, sadness, anger, and grief. Some pioneers didn't make it. They either died because of their hardships or they lived with a sad, embittered spirit until death finally relieved them.

The ones who made it are the heroes and heroines whose determination gave birth to the American spirit. It was that determination, born of faith and belief, which would have caused Edward to say to Martha:

"Martha, we have lost four babies, but many of our neighbors have suffered likewise. We can't bring them back. By constantly grieving we are causing sadness in our lives, in our children's lives, and in our friends lives. We must live for what we have. We have three healthy, happy, loving, wonderful children. The farm is finally able to feed us all adequately. I have just heard of a new crop that thrives in a soil like ours. I'm going to plant it this spring. If it thrives we'll have food for us and enough to sell. Then we can begin to buy things we've needed and even a few things we've just wanted. The children will have store-bought toys next Christmas, Martha. And you will have a bonnet with lace. We're going to make it, Martha!"

No matter how inspired I may feel by the experiences of other people, I find it far more inspiring to realize that they survived and celebrated life in spite of great difficulty. Our ancestors did more than ride through a colorful, exciting chapter in American history. They survived horrible challenges to the human body, mind, and spirit. They picked themselves up and kept going. They obviously had a strong spiritual component to their lives.

I have derived enormous strength and inspiration from my mother. When my baby was injured I wanted to be able to give him the same strength and inspiration Mother so beautifully gave to me when I was diagnosed with diabetes. Prior to John's second surgery I clung to the memories of Mother's cheerfulness and positive conviction that everything would be fine. So, with John I was full of laughter and play. We celebrated life. However, with family, friends, and pastor I contemplated the precariousness of life. My questions brought tears instead of answers. I was afraid that perhaps I was too weak to be able to inspire my child the way Mother had inspired me.

My answer came when I gained further insight into what Mother had faced and how she actually felt at that time. She always seemed so upbeat, but she told me that when she practiced giving injections to an orange, tears streamed down her face as she imagined having to inject her little girl. That revelation amazed me because it was only a smiling and positive "sergeant of arms" (and legs and buttocks) who would march into my bedroom to give me my shot and start me on my healthy way each day. I thought it had been easy for Mother to be cheerful. I felt it even more inspiring to learn that it was not easy at all, but she had done it.

Perhaps because of the environment in which he grew, perhaps all on his own, John, with proverbial "childlike faith," discovered *his* Physician Within.

When John was three years old the surgeon told us that John would need more surgery. The graft had contracted, pulling his foot up into a 90 degree angle. The surgeon solemnly told me that although he could graft enough skin to allow John to walk and run, John would never be able to completely flex his toes. "He'll never point his toes; there simply isn't enough skin," he told me.

This time the surgeon took a full thickness of skin from John's abdomen. When the stitches were removed, John's foot was in the exact position the surgeon had told us it would be. He reminded me, "Now remember, that foot is not going to come down any farther. Creams won't help. Exercise won't help. He simply doesn't have enough skin."

We went home to ride trikes and get on with our lives. One day as John was riding his trike up a particularly steep hill, I pushed on his back to help him make it up. He looked at me and insisted, "Mom, I can do it myself." So, I let go and followed alongside him. As John worked to get up the hill, his wonderful spirit came through as he hoarsely whispered the words, "I think I can. I think I can . . ."

Several months later, we returned to the plastic surgeon for a check-up. He confirmed what we had already observed: John was able to point both toes perfectly. The surgeon's face registered real shock as he said, "There's no explanation for that!"

Ten days later as John was getting out of the bathtub, I pointed to the graft donor site on his abdomen and said, "Isn't that super, John? Your scar is fading so that you can hardly see it." John looked me straight in the eyes and said, "Mom, my body's got lots of skin, and I'm healthy!"

I told that story to a group once, and there happened to be a pediatric plastic surgeon in the audience. He approached me afterwards and told me that he wasn't at all surprised at John's healing. He said that children do not understand "never." They expect to get well. And they frequently do, in spite of all our doubts and learned realism.

There is something quite wonderful about childlike faith. A

child's limited exposure to the world has not taught them hopelessness. They live in a magical world where anything is possible.

Recall the people in your life who have inspired you with their example. If possible, talk with them. Instead of romanticizing their struggle, learn how difficult it really was, and how they survived. Compare their experiences with your own, and enrich your appreciation of the power within each of us. Again, the most helpful resources for your discovery of your Physician Within will be your own intimate experience with difficulty, emotional pain, and all of life's challenges and seeming "unfairness," all of which, when overcome, add so much to the imperfect but beautiful reality of life.

The Physician Within is a Feeling, a deeply held Conviction, Faith, Hope, Trust, Belief. Philosophy, poetry, and religion are simply attempts to put all of that into words. Inasmuch as these expressions of others' feelings succeed in describing your feelings, they reinforce and *nourish* your Physician Within. Let's explore ways of nourishing, reinforcing, and sustaining the Physician Within.

Philosophy

"To teach men how to live without certainty
and yet without being paralyzed by hesitation,
is perhaps the chief thing philosophy can still do."

Bertrand Russell

The French philosopher Albert Camus made the following observation:

In the depth of winter I finally learned that
within me there lay an invincible summer.

I love that philosophical description of the Physician Within as "an invincible summer," especially in facing the "depth of winter." Life brings us many winters. A disease is one of life's winters. The force (invincible summer) which keeps you going through the darkest hours of the harshest winter is your

Physician Within.

Literature

In great literature we find grand and inspiring thoughts. They reinforce our belief, which then nourishes our Physician Within. One of my favorite literary giants is Ralph Waldo Emerson. I find important nourishment from the following quote:

> "Whatever you do, you need courage. Whatever course you decide upon, there is always someone to tell you you are wrong. There are always difficulties arising which tempt you to believe that your critics are right. To map out a course of action and follow it to an end requires some of the same courage which a soldier needs. Peace has its victories, but it takes brave (people) to win them."

There are so many messages in our culture tempting us to believe that we cannot make it. Statistics wag a threatening finger at us. Acquaintances who have the same disease we have, die. It would be so easy to let go of our positive belief, to quit.

If someone were to ask me what it has taken to live well with diabetes, I would say Faith and Courage. Courage, of course, is overcoming fear to do something. Without fear there can be no courage. Great literature is filled with inspiring stories of courage, poetry of hope and prose to reinforce those important feelings of belief.

Another of my mentors reminded me that not *all* of philosophy and literature is inspiring. Some of it is dark and disturbing. Here is where your responsibility comes in. Choose a nourishing food for your mind and soul just as you carefully select nourishing food for your body. As the German poet Goethe so beautifully put it:

> "One ought, every day at least, to hear a little song, read a good poem, see a fine picture, and, if it were possible to

speak a few reasonable words."

Here are two more examples of the fine thoughts we can gain from literature:

Where there is great love there are always miracles. Miracles rest not so much upon faces or voices or healing power coming to us from afar off, but on our perceptions being made finer, so that for a moment our eyes can see and our ears can hear what is there about us always.

Willa Cather

The best things are nearest. Breath in your nostrils, Light in your eyes, Flowers at your feet, Duties at your hand, the Path of Right just before you. Then do not grasp at the stars, but do Life's plain, common work as it comes, certain that daily duties and daily bread are the sweetest things in life.

Robert Louis Stevenson

Religion

Religion is another helpful resource to define and nourish our spiritual side. Millions of people throughout the world find their greatest power in the context of religious faith. Though so many people profess a belief in a power greater than themselves, there are many different interpretations, traditions, practices, and beliefs. I have had the most experience observing Christian faith and the *personal* relationship people speak of having with the Lord.

A woman with lupus described how the Lord had worked as her Physician Within. She told me that it was a terribly traumatic time in her life. She had just lost her husband and the stress of that caused a dreadful flare-up of her lupus. She knew that she would have to work to support her three children. But, her lupus had worsened so much that her doctor could not give her much encouragement about her future. He was concerned by how rapidly her health was declining. She knew already that her Physician Within was her ultimate hope, but now she also felt He was her *only* hope.

She went home and picked up her Bible. She turned to Hebrews. In Hebrews 12:12 she read:

"Therefore lift your drooping hands and strengthen your weak knees, and make straight paths for your feet, so that what is lame may not be put out of joint but rather be healed." She told me that she found a tremendous sense of peace and strength from that passage. She began to heal. She is now in remission. The scripture passage had sparked and reinforced her belief, which in turn activated her Physician Within.

How do you define and describe your Physician Within? If your discovery is still incomplete, then keep searching. Philosophy, literature, and religion can not only nourish and reinforce your spirit, they can also help you to discover it. Besides these resources, talk with advisors whom you respect: health professionals, clergy, educators, friends you admire, and any people you know who are "survivors" in the best sense of the word: they have made the best of what they've been given in life, may it be poverty, injury, illness, or chronic disease. If you seek your spirit with the belief in your heart that you will find it ... you will. Once you discover your Physician Within, you will realize that that power has been within you all along.

Remember, the only way in which we can activate the Physician Within is through faith ... belief. It is so easy *not* to believe. Belief can be so fragile. Reality is often so bold and large and strong. A friend of mine was a guest in our home once. She is dead now. When she was last in our home she was a blind, kidney-recipient, amputeed young woman. I helped her to prepare for her bath. As I lowered her frail little body into the bath tub I grieved for her, but I also grieved for myself. Diabetes had caused all that devastation to her body. I have the same disease. Belief in health is difficult when the reality of disease is so strong. I remember quite vividly what it felt like to rub cream on the stump of her leg.

Reality's voice is shrill and piercing to the core of our being. The Physician Within must be a very powerful force in order to absorb the piercing cry of reality and answer back with calm, sure, strength: "Yes, but I am in control. Trust. Believe."

I am convinced that disease and pain and difficulty are blessings because of the spiritual growth they bring. Without struggle, we remain weak. A perfect illustration of this comes from the story of a man who raised butterflies as a hobby. He was so touched by the difficulties they had in emerging from the cocoon, that once, out of mistaken kindness, he split a cocoon with his thumbnail so that the tiny inmate could escape without a struggle. That butterfly was never able to use its wings.

To find the strength to carry on with whatever struggle life brings, you need an unending source of inner power: Your Physician Within. The times we are not aware of that power are the times when we are ignoring it. There again is the beauty of great suffering, because it is then that we seek that force. It is your responsibility to connect with your Physician Within. View it as a huge generating plant into which you must be "plugged" in order to make use of its energy and power. We can use it or not; it is our choice. If you choose to connect with this power source, look for all the "sockets" you can plug yourself into. Receive all the spark it has to ignite your spirit.

Even with an active internal power, we are not towers of strength, acceptance, and peace all of the time. There are times of honest questioning, times of vulnerability, momentary returns of anger and sadness over disease and disability. And there are simply days when we're a bit "down." These are the times to turn — with the help of our Physician Within—to our external power sources and receive their spark.

Sparks to Ignite Your Spirit

If religion is the basis of your spirit, then it is the teaching of your faith that will ignite and sustain you spiritually. Some of my favorite passages from the Bible are: Hebrews 10:35,36; Philippians 4:6,7 and 11-13; Isaiah 26:3; Joshua 1:9; and John 16:33. Seek your own and keep a list. Let me share one passage:

> "We rejoice in our sufferings, knowing that suffering produces endurance, and endurance produces character and character produces hope, and hope does not disappoint us."

Romans 5:3-5

People can be wonderful sparks. This book is "peopled" by the brave men and women from my world as I have observed them and been inspired by them. Look for these inspiring people in your life. They're there.

> One of my dearest friends has been an inspiring model to me all my life. Norma is 92 years old as this book is being written. During the Depression Norma and her husband owned and managed a hotel. Harry became very ill and required round-the-clock nursing care. Norma struggled to run the hotel all by herself.

> One day I asked Norma, "How did you make it?" She responded with the spirit of practicality and faith that I have admired in so many people. "Well, on days when I was feeling down I'd think about someone worse off than I. Then, I'd go visit them. On days when I was really down I'd go to a movie where I could escape for a couple of hours. Feeling refreshed I would then visit someone in a nursing home or hospital. Then, I'd get on with my life."

Nature is a magnificent spark! Have you ever looked so closely at a Norway pine tree that it stirred a feeling of inspiration in you? The Norway pine is tall, straight, strong, resolute, yet able to bend and sway with the wind. What a lesson we can learn from this beautiful, resilient tree!

Mother Nature shared some of her inspiration with me through birds. One April we had a blizzard in Minnesota. The robins in our neighborhood had already built their nests, and the blizzard destroyed them. I saw that the robins did not give up. They rebuilt their nests. What resilience and determination!

I read a story once in which a bird's nest was robbed of its young by a predator. The forest was momentarily silent. Then, the birds began to sing again. Even this simple creature seems to realize that life is for the living. We must go on. What a lesson in faith.

When Notre Dame football coach Lou Holtz was coach at the University of Minnesota, he shared a story with the same message. He said that the greatest halfback he ever coached was not great because he never got knocked down. He was great because he never stayed down!

Music was mentioned in the stress management chapter as a means to help us relax. It can also serve as a spark. People in the music world often adopt a musical "signature," a song with which they are identified. Henry Mancini's signature is "The Stripper," a song which obviously stirs and inspires him. The late Arthur Fiedler's was "The Stars and Stripes Forever." Can you imagine the feeling he must have had each time he heard that rousing, charged up music? Identify music that does that for you, and play it, sing it, really participate in it.

Art is another fine resource for spiritual nourishment. I cannot recommend specific works of art, for the beauty in art is in each individual's interpretation and enjoyment of it. Visit an art gallery or museum. Be open to receiving not only a message from works of art, but also a feeling of inspiration. I will never forget seeing a statue of Joan of Arc in the Cathedral of Notre Dame in Paris. The feeling I got as I looked at that beautiful statue was the feeling of great peace and strength in the face of great adversity and pain. Many years later I met a wonderful woman who reminded me of that work of art and its inspiring message. The woman has painful and crippling arthritis throughout her entire body. But, when one looks into her face, one never sees pain, only peace and gentle strength.

A photograph can inspire. A friend of mine who is a cardiologist recommends exercise to his patients not only for the physiological benefit, but also for the spiritual benefit. He believes that one of the most important benefits of exercise is that it increases our self-esteem. In his lectures he uses a slide showing a woman running up a hill. Superimposed on the picture are the words: "The Sound of Cheering from Within." Surely it is her Physician Within who is doing that cheering. I love that picture and I love my friend for sharing it.

Newspapers are not always full of the world's problems. The Wall Street Journal periodically has a full page sponsored by United Technologies Corporation, and rather than an advertisement, each page shares a stimulating thought. I saved the following one because it gave me a "spark."

Brighten Your Corner

Have you

noticed the

great difference

between the

people you meet?

Some are as

sunshiny as

a handful of

forget-me-nots.

Others come on

like frozen mackerel.

A cheery, comforting

nurse can

help make a

hospital stay

bearable.

An upbeat secretary

makes visitors
glad they came
to see you.
Every corner of the
world has its clouds,
gripes, complainers,
and pains in the
neck—because many
people have
yet to
learn that
honey works better
than vinegar.
You're in control
of your small
corner of the
world.
Brighten it . . .
You can.

Even a greeting card can be a spark. I love the cards by Flavia. I bought one with this message:

"Hope, like love transcends
all time. It is a friend,
a healer, a maker of dreams."

Movies can be a source of inspiration. Star Wars captured the imagination of millions of people all over the world. We learned about the "force." It was presented as a sort of energy field, a positive power that gave Luke Skywalker extraordinary power, but only if he trusted in it. The Physician Within?

Perhaps the greatest spark we can receive occurs when we are giving of ourselves to others. Dr. Hans Selye called it "altruistic egotism," because he realized that we help ourselves when we help others. It is through giving that we receive. It is the spark of your spirit touching my spirit that ignites the most powerful force in the universe: Love. I saw a banner once that said:

> Someday after mastering the winds and gravity,
>   We shall harness for God the energy of Love
>   and then for the second time in history,
>   we shall have discovered Fire.

Paul Tillich, a theologian, gave us insight into this when he said that God is not a benevolent cloud in the sky, separate from all of us "down here." Instead, God is as close as the closest human being is to us. He is in each of us and we connect with Him whenever we communicate a loving message to anyone around us. When we give or receive those loving messages we experience feelings of warmth and goodness as our Physician Within awakens and stirs. We nourish our spirit whenever, out of love, we:

* say a kind word,

* share a beautiful thought,

* telephone a friend to see how she is,

* bring soup to a neighbor in need,

* spend time with a lonely or hurting person,

* give food, clothing, or money to those in need,

* volunteer our time or talent to a worthy cause,

* hug someone,

* help someone you'll probably never see again, (a stranger in the grocery store, a child thousands of miles away),

* or . . . (continue with your own list).

Perhaps, like me, you will find that there is a lot of overlapping as you think of your Physician Within. See that overlapping as reinforcement. God is surely my invincible summer, my undying song of Hope, and my loving, healing Physician Within.

What is yours? It's there, my friend. Within you there lies abundant power to help you make it through any challenge you encounter. Find it. Nourish it. Most importantly, Believe in it!

Summary

* What is the Physician Within? It is hope that never stops, a force that lets you persevere in the face of life's most difficult and "unfair" challenges, and a peace that lets you find joy in what could be your most crushing moment. It is within everyone, but it must be discovered, realized, explored, and most of all, believed in.

* Inspiration for your belief in your Physician Within can come from the experiences of others who have survived against great odds. Seek those people out or read about them, but be realistic rather than romantic in your interpretation of their heroism. Reality is dealing with day to day routines and experiences, withstanding the drudgery and the tragedy, while fully appreciating the beauty and the joy.

* The ultimate inspiration for your belief will come from your own experiences; from experiencing peace and security at a time of great stress and uncertainty; from trusting that there is a power greater than you, which if believed in and empowered with all the faith in your heart, will be your greatest source of strength.

* Philosophy, literature, and religion can nourish your belief in your Physician Within. Seek inspiration in the thoughts of others, interpreting their ideas and expressions and applying them to your life.

* It is your responsibility to define your Physician Within. If you are not already aware of that force, explore the sense of inner strength others place their faith in. Then look back on your life, and examine your current situation. Search for that force with the belief that you will find it, because it is there.

Reflection Questions

1. Describe your Physician Within.

2. When do you most feel the presence of this force?

3. Describe how you call on it for help when you need it. Is it always there for you?

4. List the ways in which you connect with your Physician Within.

Make Your
Plan of Action!

The end of this book signals the beginning of your journey. See your progress toward wellness along the minus 100 to plus 100 continuum. You may experience one of the many mud slides of life, which will bring you to the left, and possibly back to zero or worse. That's where perseverance comes in. Get back on track. Pick up your coping tools and use them to take control. Move yourself in the direction of total well-being (plus 100) by using all the skills presented in this book:

   Choosing a wellness approach to every challenge
   Building a positive self-image
   Motivating yourself to maintain healthy behaviors and a
   hopeful outlook
   Adapting to life's constantly changing circumstances
   Managing stress with positive coping techniques
   Finding solutions to your problems
   Activating your support system
   Knowing that your Physician Within will keep you going

Now, put all of these skills together to design your "Plan of Action." Your plan begins with a goal, which in broad terms is "to live well." You must give that statement your own special and specific meaning.

The next step is to include as many healthy lifestyle behaviors as are appropriate to your goal and your health situation. These behaviors both protect and enhance your life. They are really no different than those recommended for everyone, which reinforces the fact that our goal is to be well. In spite of the limitations of a disease or disability, everyone can participate in some healthy behaviors. Examples include such things as wearing seatbelts, eating nutritious meals, exercising regularly, managing stress through positive coping techniques, daily rest and relaxation, and taking regular vacations. What others would you add? In listing your healthy behaviors in your plan of action, be as specific as possible so that you will be able to evaluate your progress.

If you have special needs, there will be additional healthy behaviors that you will want to follow. These can include specific exercises, physical therapy, a particular meal plan, medication, or various other treatments to enhance your well-being.

Because you are human you will encounter obstacles. It can help to reflect ahead of time on what you think those obstacles might be. Some may be related to your challenge or its treatment. Pain may make your prescribed exercise difficult. The effects of chemotherapy may make positive thinking seem like an impossibility. Obstacles related to your humanness include unresolved anger (I'm not going to take care of this disease. I don't want it!"), lack of motivation ("I know I 'should' do this, but . . ."), discouragement ("I can't keep going. It's more than I can take.") and many, many others. Be realistic in identifying your obstacles.

Your understanding of your own well-being will help you to overcome your obstacles. Use the process described in the Solution Finding chapter.

Finding support will also help you overcome obstacles. Your Plan of Action needs lots of support so that you have the necessary encouragement and motivation. List your external supports - your sources of help and encouragement, and describe your internal support - your source of faith.

Include a reward system in your plan. Promise yourself a reward for following the healthy behaviors you have set for yourself.

Finally, know your distress signs. What signs tell you that you are headed down the wrong path? Missing your doctor appointments? Skipping exercise sessions? Forgetting to take your medication? Dwelling on negative thoughts? Feeling sorry for yourself? These are all one-way signs pointing to the minus 100 on the wellness continuum. After identifying your signs of distress, determine where you will go to get the support or the boost you need to get yourself going again in the right direction. The following pages contain several blank Plans of Action. Fill one in for yourself right now. Then, use the others whenever you feel a need to get your life back in balance, focused on wellness. Also, share them - and this book - with others who could benefit.

Your Plan of Action is your personalized road map, leading to a happy, healthy, fulfilling life. We are travelers, you and I. Our destinations may be different. Our detours will be different. But our purpose is the same: to live well. It is not disease that brings us together. It is our desire and hope for wellness.

I close with another "spark," and I wish you well.

We are all travelers.
From "birth to death,"
we travel between the eternities.
May these days be
pleasant for you, profitable for society,
Helpful to those you meet, and a Joy
to those who know and love you best.

Plan of Action

My Goal is to live well. To me this means:

In order to reach my goal of a fulfilling life I will follow these healthy lifestyle behaviors:

regular exercise, nutritious eating habits, effective stress management, regular vacations, and:

Because I have special needs I will also follow these healthy behaviors:

Obstacles which I may encounter include:

I will overcome these obstacles by:

To keep my battery charged along the way I will receive encouragement, motivation, and support from the following exciting activities, inspirational readings, loving advisors, and loyal friends:

When I successfully follow the healthy, positive behaviors (including my choice of positive, constructive thoughts) I will reward myself with:

My distress signs are:

When I notice a distress sign I will turn for support to:

EPILOGUE

Now, friends, it is your turn to take the ideas discussed in this book and expand upon them. Use them in the laboratory of life. It is then that you will discover which tools are useful in your life and which additional tools are necessary in order for you to build a healthy mind, body and spirit.

Please write and share your discoveries. Your input will be very valuable as we continue to create tools for Health Professionals and the clients who have health challenges. The DCI Wellness Series is working on the development of the Health Professional complement to this book. Its working title is:*Motivation for Healthy Living: The Health Professional's Role.* Another project is a motivational video. Let us know the tools you would find useful.

Whether you are a health professional (physical, mental or spiritual), client or concerned friend please join in this exciting quest to find those paths which lead to Well-Being. Send your insights to me at:

Catherine Feste
care of Diabetes Center, Inc.
P.O. Box 739
Wayzata, MN 55391

Plan of Action

Use this abbreviated Plan of Action for achieving less complex goals.

A specific, measurable description of my goal is:

I will use the following healthy behaviors to work toward my goal:

I will use the following coping strategies when I encounter obstacles:

My reward(s) for following the healthy behaviors will be:

Plan of Action

Use this abbreviated Plan of Action for achieving less complex goals.

A specific, measurable description of my goal is:

I will use the following healthy behaviors to work toward my goal:

I will use the following coping strategies when I encounter obstacles:

My reward(s) for following the healthy behaviors will be:

Plan of Action

Use this abbreviated Plan of Action for achieving less complex goals.

A specific, measurable description of my goal is:

I will use the following healthy behaviors to work toward my goal:

I will use the following coping strategies when I encounter obstacles:

My reward(s) for following the healthy behaviors will be:

If you found this book helpful and would like more information on this and other related subjects you may be interested in one or more of the following titles from our *Wellness and Nutrition Library.*

BOOKS:

The Joy of Snacks — Good Nutrition for People Who Like to Snack
(288 pages)
The Physician Within (210 pages)
Pass The Pepper Please (90 pages)
Fast Food Facts (40 pages)
Convenience Food Facts (137 pages)
Opening The Door To Good Nutrition (186 pages)
Learning To Live Well With Diabetes (392 pages)
Exchanges For All Occasions (210 pages)
A Guide To Healthy Eating (60 pages)

BOOKLETS & PAMPHLETS

Diabetes & Alcohol (4 pages)
Diabetes & Exercise (20 pages)
Emotional Adjustment To Diabetes (16 pages)
Healthy Footsteps For People With Diabetes (13 pages)
Diabetes Record Book (68 pages)
Diabetes & Brief Illness (8 pages)
Diabetes & Impotence: A Concern for Couples (6 pages)
Adding Fiber To Your Diet (10 pages)
Gestational Diabetes: Guidelines for A Safe Pregnancy and Healthy Baby
(24 pages)
Recognizing and Treating Insulin Reactions (4 pages)
Hypoglycemia (functional) (4 pages)

The *Wellness and Nutrition Library* is published by Diabetes Center, Inc. in Minneapolis, Minnesota, publishers of quality educational materials dealing with health, wellness, nutrition, diabetes and other chronic illnesses. All our books and materials are available nationwide and in Canada through leading bookstores. If you are unable to find our books at your favorite bookstore contact us directly for a free catalog:

Diabetes Center, Inc.
P.O. Box 739
Wayzata, MN 55391